Praise for *Mercies in Disguise*

"A moving, suspenseful page-turner that's likely to become a classic of medical storytelling."　　—*The Washington Post*

"Absorbing . . . the interweaving tales of science, family, and medical ethics make for a compelling read."
　　　　　　　　　　　　　　—*Library Journal*

"Gripping . . . Kolata's book reads like a medical thriller."
　　　　　　　　　　　　　　—*Publishers Weekly*

"A story that pits hope against fate, courage against uncertainty . . . Kolata delivers an inspiring chronicle of a remarkable family, medical advances, and redefining destiny."　　—*Booklist*

"*Mercies in Disguise* is the true story of one family's struggle with a rare and deadly inherited illness. Gina Kolata's prose brings to life the science as well as the maverick scientists who solve the riddle. When a blood test can now predict who is destined to be an invalid while still young, and who is spared, we agonize with family members over whether we'd want such knowledge. *Mercies in Disguise* reads like a medical thriller; I simply couldn't stop once I began."
　　　　　　　—Dr. Abraham Verghese, author of the
　　　　　　　*New York Times* bestseller *Cutting for Stone*

"*Mercies in Disguise* is an extraordinary medical mystery, scientific history, and, above all, human drama. Once I started reading, I couldn't stop. Then, when I finished it, I couldn't stop thinking about the Baxleys and the choices they faced."
　　—Sylvia Nasar, author of *A Beautiful Mind,* winner of the
　　　　National Book Critic̓s Circle Award for Biography

## ALSO BY GINA KOLATA

*Rethinking Thin*

*Ultimate Fitness*

*Flu*

*Clone*

*Sex in America*
(with Robert T. Michael,
John H. Gagnon,
Edward O. Laumann)

*The Baby Doctors*

# Mercies in Disguise

*A Story of Hope,*
*a Family's Genetic Destiny,*
*and the Science That*
*Rescued Them*

Gina Kolata

ST. MARTIN'S GRIFFIN
NEW YORK

*To Amanda and the Baxley family*

www.stmartins.com

The Library of Congress has cataloged the hardcover edition
as follows:

Names: Kolata, Gina Bari, 1948– author.
Title: Mercies in disguise : a story of hope, a family's genetic
    destiny, and the science that rescued them / Gina Kolata.
Description: First edition. | New York : St. Martin's Press,
    2017. | Includes bibliographical references and index.
Identifiers: LCCN 2016044044 | ISBN 9781250064349
    (hardcover) | ISBN 9781250123992 (ebook)
Subjects: LCSH: Medical genetics. | Genetic disorders. |
    Genetic screening—Moral and ethical aspects. | BISAC:
    MEDICAL / Genetics. | HEALTH & FITNESS / Diseases /
    Genetic. | BIOGRAPHY & AUTOBIOGRAPHY /
    Medical. | SCIENCE / Life Sciences / Genetics &
    Genomics.
Classification: LCC RB155.5 .K65 2017 | DDC 616/.042—dc23
LC record available at https://lccn.loc.gov/2016044044

ISBN 978-1-250-06444-8 (trade paperback)

Our books may be purchased in bulk for promotional,
educational, or business use. Please contact your local
bookseller or the Macmillan Corporate and Premium Sales
Department at 1-800-221-7945, extension 5442, or by email at
MacmillanSpecialMarkets@macmillan.com.

First St. Martin's Griffin Edition: March 2018

D   10  9  8  7  6  5

# Contents

# Contents

The two most important days in your life are the
day you are born and the day you find out why.

—MARK TWAIN

What if trials of this life
The rain, the storms, the hardest nights
Are your mercies in disguise?

—"Blessings," BY LAURA STORY

# Introduction

The two people Amanda Baxley loves the most begged her not to be tested—at least not now. "Please," her mother pleaded. "Your dad is so sick. We are hurting so much already." Her boyfriend implored her not to invite news that could cast such a long and dark shadow over their future. "You don't know what it will do to you," he warned.

But she had always been so stubborn, so sure of what she wanted, so able to push past trepidation. And she was driven by the impossible expectations of what this day would bring; she had to know her future in order to control it. If she had the mutated gene—a forecast of a horrifying and fatal illness, one without treatment or cure, passed down in her family from generation to generation—she vowed it would stop with her.

So today, with her mother and boyfriend beside her for support, Amanda sits across from her therapist—a man she first saw when she was in college, when her troubles with her boyfriend seemed overwhelming. Now, at twenty-six years old, she is facing a dilemma that seems to reach beyond her young adulthood, into the ageless realm of the surreal. *Which life will it be?* The one in which the years stretch outward boundlessly or the one where the future twists into a discernible, ghastly shape? Amanda glances around the room. The office is as it ever was: cozy with a fireplace across from a love seat and a couple of chairs. She has been here many times before, but now it is another world.

A gamine with huge brown eyes and short, glossy brown hair, Amanda vibrates with energy. And though she isn't able to bring it to bear at this particular moment, she is an optimist, always reaching instinctively for promise. She's a hugger and a weeper, someone who does not hide her emotions. Today, she is still glowing from a recent trip to Africa, where she was able to forget herself a little while helping people who had so much less than she. At times, she was even able to forget this day, persuade herself it was not coming, this moment that will inextricably change her life.

Amanda's fate resides in the result of a blood test. It will reveal whether she possesses a single mutated gene, one that has contorted the fates of so many of her family members. The results are with a doctor in California, who'd ordered the test. In a few minutes the phone will ring and that doctor, on the other side of the country, will open the envelope and tell her, over speakerphone, the fateful news.

If your family carried a mutated gene that foretold a brutal illness and you were offered the chance to find out if you'd inherited it, would you do it? Would you walk toward the problem, bravely accepting whatever answer might come your way? Or would you turn away, hoping to protect yourself from knowing too much?

Testing would allow you to prepare; it would permit you to plan your life accordingly, tying up loose ends and making adjustments for your truncated future. It would be practical. Perhaps it would feel the only responsible thing to do: to tell your partner or spouse that he or she will be bound to this illness, as you are. It might keep you from passing your fate on to unborn children. On the other hand, divining this illness could rob you of the limited number of carefree years left to you—years that could be spent pursuing a life you'd once taken for granted. Perhaps choosing not to know would allow you to retain a certain innocence, hopefully preserving a part of the person you were before being faced with such a dilemma. Were you to choose to live in ignorance, though, you might remain peripherally alert to the first signs of fatality: a slackening grip or a spasm in a muscle. But then, we all know the rough outline—there is the certitude of death for everyone—so why take on the weight of learning the specifics? What would you do with this information, knowing there is nothing you can do to stop the illness?

This is the story of an almost archetypal family in a small town in South Carolina faced with a medical mystery they were determined to solve.

The Baxley family is a proud and determined clan, including among them respected doctors, dignified in their approach. They are a family that works hard to maintain a close-knit bond. Though they experienced the usual abrasions—teenage rebellions, angst over career choices, personality clashes—overall, life was good.

Until, without warning, they were thrust into a harrowing medical dilemma. One by one, various members of the family were struck with an inscrutable disease, made more perplexing by the fact that it changed form slightly with each new person who got it. Often it started with a dizzy feeling or a bit of confusion. This progressed to shaky hands that could not hold a pen and moved on to lurching movements of the body. The disease ultimately rendered its victims unable to talk or to swallow without choking. And it always ended in death.

Doctors, even specialists at leading medical centers, were perplexed. The disease mimicked some of the physical symptoms of Parkinson's and some of the neurological symptoms of Alzheimer's—and yet this illness exists entirely in its own sphere.

For a brief and intertwining period of history, the scientific world and the Baxley family found themselves on parallel missions to unlock the mystery of this illness.

The scientific quest began with diseases like none the researchers had ever seen before. Their very nature seemed to violate the laws of biology. This class of disease was infectious but could also be inherited through mutated genes. But the principal hypothesis for why this would be true—substantiated in studies and experiments—was fiercely rejected by many prominent researchers. Gradually, however, the pieces fell into place and that once crazy-sounding hypothesis, involving distorted proteins and gene mutations that can produce them, gained credence. The revelations were so groundbreaking that two Nobel Prizes—separated by nearly thirty years—were awarded to the lead researchers. And though the Baxleys had not yet discovered it, their family was carrying one of those mutated genes.

As these two tales converged—scientific and familial—they brought to light a fatal gene mutation and a blood test that could reveal who had it. Now the Baxleys could know who in the family had inherited this curse—and who would be spared.

This is a story of a family that took matters into its own hands when the medical world abandoned them. It is a story of how science presented the Baxley family members with a responsibility they'd never asked for or anticipated—but that each took on in their own daring way. And it is a story of how a horrific disease taught a family forbearance and the ability to find hope even as the daunting circumstances threatened to extinguish it. This is a story of disrupting destiny.

*  *  *

In her therapist's office, Amanda is on edge, suddenly wondering if perhaps she has mistaken headstrong for thoughtful; this *was* what she had wanted when she sent in the vial of her blood for the test, wasn't it? She thought she'd been doing the hard work to prepare herself all along, but suddenly it feels as if there are no laws—physical, moral, or otherwise—nothing to hold her to the ground, no promise that it will be all right, no map to guide her afterward.

The phone rings. The California doctor is on the line.

"Are you ready, Amanda?" her therapist asks.

*Part I*

# A Disease

# Prologue

They called it *kuru*—"to be afraid" or "to shiver." It was identified by its early symptoms—wobbling legs and a distinctive tremor that spread steadily through the limbs. Before long the victim's whole body would begin to shake constantly and uncontrollably. Shaking would turn to flailing, and flailing to a loss of muscle control that invariably left the patient unable to stand or walk or even sit without assistance. The tongue would become flaccid, unresponsive, so words were slurred, speech was incomprehensible. Facial muscles would twitch, pulling the visage into a series of exaggerated expressions. And then, after about five months, all movement would suddenly cease: the face frozen into an unblinking mask from which two eyes stared wildly, reflecting the increasingly disoriented mind of a person descending into mute dementia. Death would follow soon after.

No one had ever been known to recover from kuru and its symptoms. The affliction always ran the same relentless course and it was found only among the Fore, a small group of people living in the eastern highlands of New Guinea. They thought the disease was caused by sorcery: a curse they'd lived with for decades.

The Fore population, about ten thousand individuals, slept in low grass huts in small communities clustered throughout

9

the highlands. The men—who subsisted primarily on the animals they hunted—almost always lived apart from the women and children. In the 1950s, when our story begins, they lived presumably as they had since the dawn of their time; to a Western eye, it seemed as if they had been preserved in a time capsule, sealed off from other tribes as well as from everyone else in the outside world.

This complete isolation wasn't a coincidence or community choice—it was a condition imposed upon them by their neighbors, an extended quarantine enforced from outside. The surrounding peoples had pushed the Fore back behind Kuru ("trembling") Mountain—the only time in known history that a mountain has been named for a disease—in an attempt to keep the illness in place. They too believed sorcery could spread the disease and wanted no part of it. As for the outside world, who would set out to travel through the wild rain forests in territory rumored to be inhabited by violent people, even cannibals?

Though no one had made the connection, kuru was not as unique as it appeared. Strange diseases that resembled it had been cropping up for centuries throughout the world. These illnesses often took hold of entire families. They would show up in a parent, in siblings, in aunts and uncles and cousins, generation after generation. But these diseases were so rare, and so inexplicable, that they were mentioned only in obscure medical journals. Without a clue as to what was causing the disease, or what to do about it, the world turned away.

# 1

# The Prophecy

Tim Baxley never even got the name of the woman who told him the story that set the horror in motion. It was a June evening in 1998 and Tim was at the end of the receiving line at a viewing the night before a funeral—his father's funeral.

Tim's father, Bill Baxley, had been a chemical engineer at a local packaging plant. Tall and imposing, with a stern and serious face, he had been a deacon in his church and head of the Sunday school program. He was known in his community as a problem solver, someone whom people would go to for advice or solace.

The Baxley family had lived in or near Hartsville, South Carolina, for generations. A town that, with its suburbs, comprises twenty-one thousand people and sixteen churches—eight of which are Baptist—but not a single mosque or synagogue, it is a deeply Christian population in the heart of the Bible Belt.

The lure of the town, its magnetic appeal for the Baxley family and many others, is its sense of community. Residents frequent family-owned stores because they like to buy from people they know. They support the town's free medical clinic, funded by churches, foundations, businesses, and individuals and staffed by volunteer doctors and nurses who treat those who cannot afford to pay. They cherish family life—restaurants close on Sunday nights so employees can eat dinner at home with their families. High school sports make front-page news in the town's paper. The church basketball teams take time-outs during the games for devotions. It is a place of conservative tradition, of exacting conformity, stifling to some but a comfort to those who have come to feel that Hartsville is their true home.

Bill Baxley proudly fit in. So staunch a patriarch and so perfect a picture of traditional southern living was he that, in 1985, he was awarded a plaque from Governor Richard Riley naming his clan South Carolina Family of the Year "in recognition of the exemplary qualities of family life exhibited by the William H. Baxley, Jr. family."

It was a confirmation of Bill's belief, shared by his family, that the Baxley clan was special, maybe even indestructible—certainly a testament to the grace conferred by faith, discipline, and hard work. Even Bill's viewing at the funeral home seemed to confirm this belief.

Tim knew the respect his father commanded, yet he was still astonished by the size of the crowd that night. The viewing was supposed to start at 6:00 p.m. and end at 8:00, but people lined up outside the door at 5:45. The last did not leave until 10:00. Hundreds arrived—more than the funeral director had ever seen—a steady stream of people coming despite the thick heat of that June evening. The line snaked around the wall on the right side of the front room of the funeral home, then extended out the door and through the parking lot and down the sidewalk. The family formed its own small line in that front room, greeting people as they came by. Bill Baxley lay in an open casket in a small room just behind them. Many could not bear to see him—they left after paying their respects to the family. Others, as is the Baptist tradition, filed past the casket, with no kneeling, no signs of the cross, just a solemn acknowledgment of the revered man.

The Baxley men were readily identified by strong, dark brows shading large, dark eyes, a head of thick chestnut hair, a narrow oval face and a straight, angular nose. They all had a sensuously full upper lip with a pronounced Cupid's bow. From generation to generation, the Baxley boys looked so similar that it was difficult at times to tell them apart.

But this man in the casket—this man looked nothing like Bill Baxley. He was a stranger. A rippled sateen pillow tipped a shriveled face up to the line of passing mourners. Bill's gray hair had been pulled back, the skin drawn tight against his forehead. Heavy makeup was smeared over the scar where his brain had been removed in a vain attempt to figure out the illness that had robbed him of his life. His favorite charcoal gray suit hung loose on his shrunken body; his red tie with a South Carolina emblem did nothing to draw the eye from the desolation of his body.

Tim was at the front of the receiving line, standing ahead of his older brothers, Billy, Mike, and Buddy. He glanced back at his mother—tiny, frail-looking Merle—who stood near the entrance to the room where her husband's casket lay. It would be a long night for her; she'd borne a heavy burden. And yet, after years of watching her commanding husband degrade into an invalid, aging twice as quickly as he should have, after years of helplessly watching as aides transferred his weight from wheelchair to toilet and back again, after spoon-feeding him his meals, after waiting while he communicated by grunting or nodding or slowly pointing to letters on an alphabet board, she felt in spite of herself a kernel of relief that his suffering was now over.

Between greeting visitors, Tim observed his mother shake

well-wishers' hands and acknowledge their sympathy. She was bearing up better than he had dared to hope. He developed a kind of rhythm. He'd accept a "sorry for your loss" with a grateful smile and then turn his head to see his mother doing the same thing.

Soon, the motions became automatic. So he paid little notice to the plump gray-haired woman from the nearby town of Darlington when she made her way up to him, one of so many in that sea of mourners.

"I am so sorry for your loss."

Now her eyes turned down, her smile faded slightly. She looked up at him again, holding his glance meaningfully.

"I remember his daddy walking through the plant. He had to hang on to the machines."

This seemingly innocuous comment was delivered so quietly that she had already moved on by the time Tim recognized its meaning.

Throughout his father's illness—abrupt in its onset and unswerving in its course—Tim Baxley had sought answers from one doctor after another—general practitioners, pathologists, neurologists. And he'd never received one that satisfied him. His father, doctors said, suffered from a rare, anomalous disease, kind of a blend of Alzheimer's and Parkinson's, but his was a case like none any of them had ever seen or heard of before. And yet, suddenly, in the briefest of exchanges, this woman had conveyed that she had seen it before in his grandfather—a crucial detail Tim had never known. That loss of balance, it was one of the first signs, wasn't it?

Standing there in the funeral home, Tim was barraged by memories and images, one after the other. His dad shuffling as he walked; soon the shuffling turned into stumbling and then a sort of weaving, like he was drunk. The way his father careened through the living room, clutching at the wall for support, hanging on to chairs and sofas. And that was in the beginning, when things just seemed off, but nothing so strange that it could suggest a fatal problem.

Bill's memory seemed to slip around this time as well. Tim had first noticed it ten years earlier, in 1988, at Sunday dinner at his parents' house. He had been looking for something in the basement when he came upon an object from his childhood. Bill had fought in the Pacific—but one of his friends, who had fought in Europe, had given him a compass that he had snagged from a German general. It had a steel case that opened to reveal the compass; on the other side, there was a little mirror with the initials of its owner etched on it.

Tim would often bring this to his father and ask him to talk about the war, to tell the story of his friend and how he came to get his hands on that compass. That night, Tim cradled the little compass in his hand, carrying it upstairs to the kitchen. He proudly showed it to his father. Like a small child, he wanted to hear his dad tell the story one more time. It had been years since he had asked him about it.

But when Bill looked down at what his son was holding, he seemed baffled and muttered that he had no idea what Tim was talking about. Tim reminded Bill that they'd looked at that compass many times over the years. No, Bill shot back, he didn't remember any of that. "I've been through several cases of burnout at work since that time," he offered as feeble defense.

Tim sadly trudged back downstairs clutching the compass and replaced it on the shelf—it may still be there to this day. He was devastated and tried to find a logical reason for his father's puzzling memory loss. Maybe it was depression, he thought. But what did his father mean when he offered that odd excuse? What was he telling Tim when he said "since that time"?

There would soon be more worrying signs of trouble.

The time Bill had been in a meeting at work and suddenly realized he had no idea what was going on. It was as if he had blacked out, yet he was fully conscious. This was the first signal that something was wrong, which he predictably kept to himself for a while. He didn't want to worry anyone. He didn't want to admit weakness. Eventually he told Merle, who kept it quiet for many years. Maybe it was nothing, she reasoned. It could happen to anyone with too much on his mind.

The day when Bill and Merle were out walking, a doctor who lived next door noticed that Bill was lagging behind, dragging his feet and walking unsteadily; he finally asked Merle if Bill was okay. He suggested that he do a physical exam. But when Merle brought Bill in, the doctor was confounded. Maybe a neurologist could figure it out?

The time Tim's older brother, Mike, drove Bill and Merle to a neighboring town. They were picking up windows for a sunroom Bill was building onto the house. They'd emptied out the station wagon, leaving the trunk clear to transport the unwieldy sheets of glass. Mike carried them from the store to the car and then waited for Bill, who had always taken charge in these kinds of situations. But instead Bill just frowned at the stack of glass, unable to figure out what to do. He had the frustrated look of someone asked to solve a puzzle beyond his abilities. Mike cringed, trying to seem unconcerned as he loaded the windows into the trunk. "Something is wrong with

Dad." Mike was the first to say it out loud, to Merle, finally speaking the words everyone had been thinking.

Bill grappling in vain with a little package of crackers at a Sunday family dinner, fighting his mounting frustration. That crinkling sound seemed never to end as Bill tried fruitlessly to tear open the plastic with his trembling hands, his weak fingers, never saying a word to his family as he furtively worked away at the wrapper. The rest of the family—the four sons, the three grandchildren—silent, staring at their plates, not wanting to embarrass him, knowing he would not accept help. Finally Mike reached over and, without asking, quietly opened the package.

The family watched with sorrow as Bill lost coordination in his hands. His speech blurred. As one scary symptom followed another, it was impossible to avoid the unthinkable. Something terrible was happening. Bill became desperate for a diagnosis, started begging for help. Could no one figure out what was causing this? His son Buddy was a doctor. Maybe he could assist. Tim remembered those Sunday dinners when Buddy arrived with his family. Bill would usher him into the back bedroom, saying he wanted Buddy's advice on what to do, how to get a diagnosis at least. But Buddy was at a loss.

And so, that same year—1988—when Bill's symptoms had become so distressing, Tim and his brothers began ferrying their father from doctor to doctor. This went on for years as his disease worsened and they sought help in an ever-widening area: Hartsville, then nearby towns, then the Medical University of South Carolina a couple of hours away. But the answer was always the same—some glorified version of "I don't know"— a strange illness with a relentless progression that made Bill Baxley stagger, grab chairs, tables, anything he could reach in the early stages when he could still walk. Eventually, it took away his ability to talk and to eat without choking. It humbled the proud man who never countenanced weakness. It was a disease like Alzheimer's—but not. He may not have remembered the compass, but he still remembered who his sons were, what his wife meant to him, how it felt when he could walk and talk and eat. It was a disease unique to Bill Baxley, the doctors said.

There must be an answer out there somewhere, Tim thought. Though the local doctors had been empathetic, it was obvious they were not going to be able to help. But what about a place where doctors specialize in rare diseases, a major medical center where researchers study mysterious illnesses? The closest place like that was Duke University, 150 miles away. The brothers conferred: they were aware of just how grave a situation their father was in. The symptoms had remained subtle for quite some time, but now—nearly eleven years after that episode when Bill did not recognize the compass from World War II—he was no longer able to stand without assistance. Buddy was a family doctor; Tim was starting a residency in neurology. But so far, their combined medical training was not helping.

When Tim and Buddy explained to their brother Mike that they were hitting a wall, he offered to take their father to Duke. Mike knew it was not going to be easy to get his father there, given his condition, but he felt he had to try.

When Mike picked Bill up at his house on Tuesday afternoon, January 21, 1997, they set off in a cold, driving rain. Bill slumped down in his seat, his face ashen, and dozed off. As it turned out, Bill had sleep apnea so every few minutes or so, he would stop breathing in the midst of rattling snores. The seconds-long silence, following a loud snore, was terrifying. Mike kept swerving as he sped down the slick highway, accidentally pulling the steering wheel every time he'd reach over to give his father a shove, checking if he was still alive.

Every little mundane thing became an ordeal. Bill had to use a bathroom. Getting him in and out of the car and to a restroom along the highway was agonizing. When they finally arrived at their hotel, Mike exhausted himself just getting his father from the car to the lobby to the room. Still, as he later told his brother Tim, he harbored a hope that it would all be worthwhile.

The next morning, Mike dressed his father in an oxblood flannel shirt, khaki pants, and a fedora, put bright white socks and black slip-on shoes on his feet. He and Bill arrived on time for their appointment at the neurological disorders clinic. When they were called to go in for Bill's exam, Mike helped his father rise from a chair and gently held him up as he walked into the exam room with tiny steps. He sat his father down in a chair, facing the neurologist. Bill sat rigid, his hands on his knees, his face stiff and expressionless except for his bulging, searching eyes.

The neurologist began to question Bill, who replied with effort, sometimes with just a single word in an almost inaudible voice as he laboriously struggled to speak. Bill tried to explain that in the last week he had become pretty much unable to walk unassisted, falling after a few unsteady steps. Then the neurologist asked Bill to try to cross his arms over his chest and stand.

He cannot possibly do that, Mike thought. He will tip over. He watched as his father attempted to comply, arms crossed over his chest, bending over and struggling to rise. Bill moved only a few inches from his seat before he collapsed back onto the chair, listing to the side, his masklike face giving no sign of the panic he must have felt.

The neurologist sat impassive in his chair, doing nothing to help. Mike stepped in, hoisting his father up just before he fell to the floor.

When the neurologist asked Bill to walk back and forth in front of the wall, Mike jumped up, helping his father stand, supporting him as he tried to walk with mincing steps. The doctor continued to sit calmly in his chair—no look of sympathy to Mike, or effort to comfort Bill.

"He seemed to be so distant from the human tragedy in front of him," Mike later explained to Tim. "He didn't have that personal empathy or sympathy. He would have let him fall."

Bill was stoic, never criticizing the doctor, never complaining. But Tim, who had followed Buddy by going to medical school and was now himself a doctor, was furious at what he saw as a major failing among those in his profession. Some doctors, he said to Mike, retreated behind a wall of dispassion when confronted with difficult-to-diagnose patients like their dad; he'd seen this happen before with his professors in medical school and occasionally among colleagues. As a student and then a doctor, he'd found it disturbing; as the son of a patient, he found it unacceptable. On top of it, Mike had made that long and difficult trip and to no avail. The expert at Duke was no more able to help than the local doctors. He even resorted to the by now all-too-familiar diagnosis: Parkinson's mixed with Alzheimer's. Their medical odyssey had come to a standstill.

The Baxley brothers—realizing they were likely not going to find a medical authority to guide them—felt compelled to do *something*, to find an answer. It was devastating to watch their father helplessly deteriorate with no authority figure in sight, no expert to guide them through these mystifying circumstances. The doctors who examined their father had only made his suffering worse with their breezy dismissal of his terrifying symptoms, with their clearly inaccurate diagnoses and lack of compassion.

Tim and Buddy—both medically trained themselves—decided they would have to take matters into their own hands.

The brothers conferred privately one day after Sunday dinner at their parents' house, devising a plan. They would get some of Bill's tissue and have it analyzed—or at the very least store it in case it could help someday to solve the mystery.

But what tissue? Bill had a neurological disorder, that was clear, so perhaps the first thing to examine would be the fluid that bathed their father's brain. There was a remote chance that Bill had a condition called normal pressure hydrocephalus; they knew about it from their medical studies, but the neurologists they'd consulted had seemed uninterested—it took too much time to test for it and the chance that Bill had it really was remote. But Buddy and Tim had time for the test—Bill was their father, after all. They could make time. And the test would easily check for the condition, even rid Bill of his symptoms if he had it. The characteristic feature of that condition is what is called a magnetic gait, which means walking like your feet are sticking to the floor so powerfully you cannot lift them, as if there are magnets in your shoes and the floor is made of metal. In this instance, if a doctor removes about a third of the fluid from a person's spinal column, the person is temporarily able to walk normally again, instantly. It was certainly worth a try, they agreed.

The two brothers explained their plan to Bill, who nodded with a blank expression, unable to talk, unable to question his sons but trusting them implicitly. Tim and Buddy drove their father to Buddy's office, propping him up as he tottered up a ramp to the back door. Slowly, they made their way to an exam room, where they helped him onto a table. It felt strange—doctors do not treat their family members, doctors do not insert needles into their own fathers. But now it had become essential, they decided, that they be doctors first, sons second.

They dressed their father in a hospital gown then bent him over, baring his rounded back. Tim stared at the rail-like ribs protruding from his father's sagging pale skin. His muscles were wasted; he looked like such an old man. He pushed these thoughts to the side, trying to be impartial, professional, trying to pretend the patient in front of him was not his father. He gave his father an extra dose of lidocaine, a numbing medication. Tim spoke to his father softly. "Dad, you are going to feel a little pressure in your back and maybe a tingle in your leg." Then, gently he slid a long needle into his father's spinal column. The fluid dripped out slowly, reminding Tim of what it must be like to tap a maple tree. Buddy left the room to care for other patients, and Bill, soothed by Tim's gentle touch, fell asleep.

After nearly an hour, it was done. Tim had collected all he safely could—40 milliliters of spinal fluid—filling four long tubes. "Dad, it's time to wake up," Tim murmured, lightly nudging his father. "Let's see how you are doing."

He and Buddy turned Bill on his side chatting with him while they waited the requisite half hour before sitting him up. The concern is that patients can get a headache if they sit up too soon after losing so much spinal fluid. Then they helped their father off the table. They were hoping for an instantaneous change when Bill woke up, a sudden ability to walk, the troubling symptoms vanished. Unlikely, yes, but possible.

As soon as they got their father off the table and onto his feet, however, Buddy and Tim knew they had failed. No change.

They did not let on their disappointment. "Let's go home and get some lunch and we'll see how you do," Tim said to Bill.

Now, at least, the brothers had a sample of their father's spinal fluid. Tim had held the tubes up to the light, looking for any discoloration, which could be a sign of rampant infection or inflammation or bleeding. Nothing. The liquid was as clear as pure spring water. But perhaps something in that fluid, some protein or chemical imbalance, might hold a clue to the disease.

They were flummoxed about what the next step should be. They didn't even know what test to request if they were to send it to a lab for analysis. They would store the fluid until they had a better idea of how to use it. They carefully placed the tubes in a freezer in Buddy's office.

Some time later they had a new idea. Maybe, the brothers thought, Bill had a storage disease, a type of rare disorder caused when cells cannot rid themselves of certain substances—each disease involves a different substance. Like normal pressure hydrocephalus, storage diseases were part of their medical school curriculum. But the diseases were so rare that neither Buddy nor Tim had seen any patients with one. They knew it was extremely unlikely that Bill had such a condition, and they knew testing for it was a real shot in the dark, but they felt they had to try. So they decided to take a little plug of skin from Bill's forearm and send it to the Medical University of South Carolina where it could be analyzed. The result would tell them if their hunch—their hope—was correct. Once again, Bill nodded his mute assent.

By that time Bill was near death, in the hospital with pneumonia. They worried they wouldn't be able to get some skin before it was too late—so they lingered in their father's room until 1:00 a.m., when all was quiet and no one else was around.

Buddy dispatched Tim to stand at the door to be sure no nurses were lurking. He couldn't bear to think how awkward it would be for a nurse to catch sight of Bill's son—even a son who was a doctor—taking a piece of skin from his father.

As Tim stood watch, Buddy numbed a small area of skin on his father's right forearm and removed a tiny slice, about a quarter-inch square. He covered the wound with a Band-Aid, and then he and Tim snuck out, Buddy holding a small sterile vial containing his father's skin, floating in a chemical fixative that would prevent it from deteriorating. They sent it to the pathology department at MUSC. And they waited.

Weeks went by. Tim asked the pathologists if they had any results. They did not. Then Buddy called to ask. "We don't know where the biopsy is," the pathologists finally admitted to the brothers. "We don't know what happened to the skin."

Nine years later, the university sent Tim a letter saying it had been found behind a storage cabinet and asking what he wanted them to do with it. By then, it was too late. Even if they had wanted to analyze the skin it would have deteriorated beyond repair.

"I remember his daddy walking through the plant. He had to hang on to the machines." The woman's words from the funeral haunted Tim. He thought of his own father—lurching through rooms, grabbing onto his sons for balance—before he died. He had to consider the possibility that whatever had killed his father wasn't unique. His dad had lasted to the respectable age of seventy-three, but his grandfather had only been forty-nine when he died. Could it have been the same disease? It certainly sounded like it.

He thought of his three brothers, Buddy, Billy, and Mike. Were they all destined to die like their father? And what about their children? If it could pass from father to son—the way other traits like the famous Baxley nose and the mouth with that Cupid's bow had been replicated from generation to generation—what might that mean, exactly? Was this written into his genes too?

## 2

# "No Goddamn Bastard on Earth Has Ever Seen a Disease like This Thing"

The brain arrived in the mail one day, along with twenty vials of human serum. It was sent by Dr. Vincent Zigas, employed by the Australian public health service and stationed in the New Guinea highlands, to a lab in Melbourne, Australia. People were dying there, out in the remote rain forest, past the cloud-shrouded mountains, where few Europeans had ever been. The cause of death was a strange disease, the likes of which the doctor had never seen. The natives called it *kuru*. Probably caused by a virus, Zigas speculated. But he had no lab. Would the Melbourne scientists test the brain and vials of serum for viruses?

But when the scientists did the usual tests—those that were used routinely in the late 1950s—injecting brain tissue and serum into fertilized eggs and the brains of newborn and adult mice—they found nothing. Not only were there no viruses, there wasn't even a clue as to what it might be.

Soon afterward, a young American doctor, Daniel Carleton Gajdusek, was on his way home to the United States after doing hepatitis research in Melbourne with his mentor, the renowned scientist Frank Macfarlane Burnet. He decided to make a last-minute detour to visit some scientists in nearby Port Moresby. When the researchers there told him about Dr. Zigas and his search for an explanation of kuru, Gajdusek was intrigued. Impulsive by nature, he decided to go see the doctor—and this disease—for himself.

What Gajdusek did not do was ask official permission for his independent medical expedition, and this was not the way things were supposed to be done. Upon learning of his mentee's plans, Burnet became furious. He had invited Gajdusek to work with him, he respected Gajdusek's intelligence, and he was used to what he saw as Gajdusek's emotional immaturity, but this breach of protocol was simply unacceptable. Gajdusek had to be stopped. He pointed out that arrangements had already been made for an Australian doctor to help Zigas. "Gajdusek is not authorized to undertake work in the kuru area," Burnet sputtered in a telephone call to a colleague. "Another American invasion," he continued. "Inform the minister by radio."

But Gajdusek was already on his way. He flew to a small airstrip, a dirt runway almost overgrown by tall grass in Kainantu, a small gold-prospecting town about twenty miles from the start of kuru territory. From there, it took a few hours for him to reach Zigas—a harrowing trip by jeep over mountains, through tropical rain forests and thickets of towering bamboo trees and sugarcane taller than Gajdusek himself. This was a region of near-constant rain, of mudslides and suffocating heat. Here, people lived in thatched-roof huts in isolated villages, a Stone Age people with no written language and little knowledge of the outside world. Both men and women wore grass skirts; their diet was made up of taro roots, bananas, and fungi.

Gajdusek was undaunted. He had no particular zeal for Western luxuries. He had already been to the valleys of the Hindu Kush, the jungles of South America, the coast and inland ranges of New Britain, and the swamps and high valleys of Papua New Guinea and Malaysia. He'd seen people with rabies, choking on saliva because they could not swallow. He'd seen victims of plague, and those shivering and burning with hemorrhagic fever. He'd seen encephalitis patients screaming in pain from terrible headaches. Now he would see kuru.

When Gajdusek arrived unannounced on March 13, 1957, Zigas was taken aback. He observed the tall, skinny, and bedraggled man before him, wearing threadbare shorts, an unbuttoned plaid shirt over a soiled T-shirt, and worn-out sneakers, his black hair in a ragged crew cut. Zigas thought Gajdusek was "one of those globetrotters, a kind of 'freelance anthropologist' looking for fertile hunting ground for whimsical studies." And he talked nonstop, hitting Zigas with a barrage of monologues and questions. Zigas was astonished when Gajdusek told him he was a doctor, with a degree from Harvard and specialty training in pediatrics and infectious diseases. And yet to Gajdusek's eyes, it was Zigas who was eccentric. He reminded Gajdusek of the comedian Danny Kaye both in his appearance and his demeanor.

Despite his misgivings, Zigas was glad to have another Westerner around. He'd arrived a few years ago, to a rudimentary hospital so filthy with dirt and splashes of red betel nut juice, spit on the walls by patients, that he had to spend weeks scrubbing to achieve even a semblance of cleanliness. Native doctors there made meaningless diagnoses of diseases that may have been serious or trivial—like "bad foot" and "bad blood." Zigas treated people with infections and injuries as best he could, but he felt so isolated, so alone out there in the mountains, that he longed for the company of another Western doctor. Many of his predecessors had become addicted to drugs or alcohol as a way to cope.

After his initial astonishment, Zigas eased into the role of Gajdusek's guide in this remote place. The two doctors treated the diseases that were treatable—a skin disease of children called yaws; ulcerating open sores; leprosy—and won wide-eyed respect from the Fore when some of their antibiotics and drugs cured diseases they attributed to sorcery. But kuru was another story. It was too powerful for the doctors' medicines, the Fore said.

And they were right.

Gajdusek saw his first kuru victims the day after he arrived. He and Zigas drove four hours in Zigas's jeep to pick up two middle-aged women, unable to walk, trembling, unable to speak or feed themselves. In a dispassionate letter to Burnet, Gajdusek described their "fixed and pained faces."

He was particularly fascinated by the children with kuru. The first one he saw was a little boy, about seven years old, who'd been carried to Zigas and Gajdusek by frightened villagers. Like the women, the child could not walk and his speech was so labored and slurred as to be almost impossible to understand. He could not feed himself. His limbs were trembling. Only a few months earlier, the villagers told Zigas and Gajdusek through an interpreter, the child had been normal and healthy, running and playing, chattering with his friends.

Gajdusek wrote to his mentor in the United States, Joseph Smadel, associate director of the National Institutes of Health, hardly able to contain his enthusiasm and his horror: "I looked at those kids and said, 'Jesus Christ. No goddamn bastard on earth has ever seen a disease like this thing. This is something, Joe. This will change the world."

Gajdusek knew of no disease so widespread in a small group, so quickly incapacitating. Kuru, he wrote to Smadel, "is so astonishing an illness that clinical description can only be read with skepticism, and I was highly skeptical until two days ago when I arrived and began to see the cases on every side."

New diseases are rare; new diseases as strange as this one were all but unheard of. If Gajdusek could claim this new disease, his name would go down in medical history, maybe even attached forever to the disease. Kuru also seemed as if it might hold the key to understanding brain diseases like Alzheimer's or Parkinson's. Gajdusek knew that if he could shed light on those, it would surely mean instant fame.

He also knew, however, that if he was to take ownership of kuru, he would have to be first to publish a paper identifying it and describing it, even if he could not explain it. He set his sights on the world's most prestigious medical journal, *The New England Journal of Medicine*.

Kuru was such a riddle, though. And his goal was to explain it, not just describe it. But how do you find the cause of a disease that leaves no trace of infection in the brain or in the victim's blood? Perhaps it was not an infection, but then what was it—a poison? Where to start? He had only the most rudimentary laboratory facilities. And the possibilities in this remote area with plants and insects, snakes and toxins, all so foreign, seemed endless.

Just the logistics of finding kuru patients—a first step in figuring out the disease—took so much time and effort. Hour upon hour traveling up steep mountain slopes by foot in driving rain to reach hidden villages. One of Gajdusek's guides became incapacitated by intense pain after his leg brushed against a stinging plant; he could not walk for hours. Gajdusek himself was tortured by cuts from the razor-sharp grasses that lined the path.

Not that Gajdusek minded: give him a strange and remote area, hot and sticky weather, a six-month-long rainy season and the constant irritation of mosquitoes and flies and snakes, and he was just fine—even happy to be there. He was known among his colleagues as a man who was oblivious to creature comfort; he was grandiose, driven, a visionary. He had an uncanny memory but was distractible, with a short attention span.

He was also very smart. "The peculiar sensation I had when first meeting him I have found described best in *The Autobiography of Alice B. Toklas*," explained one of Gajdusek's students. " 'A little bell went off in Alice's head when she first met Gertrude Stein that said, "genius." ' This is what I felt when I first met Carleton."

And he knew it: at age ten, Gajdusek had stenciled the names of twelve renowned microbiologists, the likes of Louis Pasteur and Robert Koch, on the steps leading to the attic of his house. He left the last step blank, for himself.

On this trip to New Guinea, starting the work that would make him famous, Gajdusek sought children with kuru. He had spent years treating children with infectious diseases and considered himself to have a special bond with children— something that would later prove to be his downfall as, over the years, he began bringing dozens of young boys, and some girls, back to the United States to live with him, promising them an education as they left their parents and families behind. He said later that he had adopted them, but there were no formal adoption papers. Eventually this practice would lead to troubling accusations of inappropriate behavior and, finally, prison. But, in the beginning, in the New Guinea highlands, the Fore children adored him, following him around, calling him "Docta America."

There were advantages to studying kuru in children. If there was a toxin or a microbe involved, it could not have been something they were exposed to decades ago, like shingles, for example, the excruciating nerve inflammation that can follow chicken pox forty or fifty years later. In addition, children would not have chronic diseases like Alzheimer's or Parkinson's that could complicate analyses with their own neurological symptoms.

Gajdusek began to review the possible causes of kuru. It could be a hysterical illness, like the seventeenth-century outbreak of "witchcraft" in Salem. Or it could be a genetic disease, like Huntington's. Or it could be the result of a brain inflammation caused by an infection or toxin or allergic reaction.

But every hypothesis he tested, based on everything he knew from his decade of medical practice, offered the same result: nothing.

To make matters worse, there was no equipment in his rudimentary lab. Even surgical gloves—needed for handling specimens or treating yaws—were lacking while he waited for the shipments of medical equipment he'd ordered to arrive. If kuru was caused by a microbe, he'd risk infection himself if he worked without gloves. But then, he'd worked in laboratories handling tissues infected with rabies and polio and viral encephalitis, all incurable diseases, and nobody in those labs had ever got infected. He decided to forge ahead. He knew how to be careful when handling possibly infectious tissues and examining patients. He'd be safe, he told himself, rashly ignoring the real risk he was taking.

The first step was to try, in a hit-or-miss way, every possible therapy he and Zigas had on hand. They administered an antibiotic, chloramphenicol, to three children and the two middle-aged women he'd met soon after he arrived. If kuru was caused by a bacterial infection, it would clear up quickly the way a strep throat gets better when a person takes penicillin. But there was no change. In truth, Gajdusek had not really expected an antibiotic to work with a disease so unlike any bacterial infection he'd encountered or read about. But he had to work by a process of elimination.

Next, they gave another group of kuru victims phenobarbital, an epilepsy drug. They thought perhaps it might at least quell the tremors. But again, no effect.

They tried aspirin—it might tamp down any inflammation—

and vitamins B and C, and fish oil. They improved their patients' diets. Nothing.

After weeks of experimenting, the only thing Gajdusek and Zigas had to show for their efforts were more kuru victims. Gajdusek sent a pleading letter to Port Moresby's director of public health, Roy Scragg, asking if he could send any or all of the following: tranquilizers that might affect the neurological symptoms; drugs like cortisone or antihistamines that might squelch immune reactions; testosterone (a wild guess, particularly since kuru's preferred victims were women); and other types of anticonvulsants. He got them all—and still no changes.

Gajdusek even requested to have two girls, ages eight and ten, who were in the early stage of the disease sent to Australia, where, he thought, first-world medical facilities might make the difference. They are "completely cooperative, friendly, and easily manageable," he wrote in a letter to Scragg, pleading their case. "Most important now is *haste*," he wrote, "for one case is now at the *earliest recognizable stage*—a really hard thing to find." Nothing came of his suggestion—the children were not sent to Australia.

Perhaps kuru was caused by a virus that had entered the area when Europeans first came to New Guinea. If it was a virus the Fore people had never encountered, it might devastate them much the way smallpox devastated Native Americans. But no—kuru had first appeared among the Fore around 1920. And the first European to enter the area, Ted Ubank, a gold prospector, did not arrive until 1936.

Gajdusek, for all his boundless energy, was no closer to an answer. He was trying to care for kuru patients, feeding those who could no longer eat, while also doing spinal taps and collecting blood and urine and keeping up with his various scientific investigations.

Gajdusek began to reach for more eccentric explanations. Cannibalism? This would explain the gender imbalance of the illness: a full two-thirds of the children with kuru were girls; in adulthood, the ratio of women to men with kuru was 14 to 1. Fore men typically got protein by eating the animals they'd hunted, whereas women and children got by on spiders and other insects—and by eating dead relatives. Cannibalism was part of Fore funeral ceremonies, which were conducted by women and children, usually girls. Could it be that kuru was present in the brains and organs of its victims and spread when they were eaten? Or, more likely, during those funeral ceremonies, as the Fore touched the organs and brains of kuru victims and then rubbed their eyes or scratched a bite on their skin, did they infect themselves? It would be easier to spread a disease that way than for a microbe to survive digestion in the stomach and then make its way to the brain. But there was no sign of an infection, so what was being transmitted?

He then turned to the idea that a toxin caused kuru. But again he and Zigas hit a dead end. They found nothing unusual in the dyes the Fore used to paint their skin or the smoke they breathed from their fires. Nothing in their diets. Nothing in their blood, urine, cerebrospinal fluid, or tissues obtained at autopsy. If there was a toxin, Gajdusek admitted, it would have to be "mighty unusual to explain why 15 women got the disease for every man."

"What is urgently needed is expert neuropathology of an entire well-fixed brain," Gajdusek wrote once again to Scragg, "with all types of staining techniques and long-term intensive study." The pathological exam could reveal areas of destruction in the brain that might explain the symptoms of kuru and give hints about what sort of disease or poison might be causing the disease. But if there was a new virus, for example, destroying the brain, staining would not show it.

Gajdusek could try to get a brain from someone who died of kuru—though this would not be easy given how carefully the Fore guarded body parts, believing sorcerers could use them to cast evil spells.

Gajdusek had to know, he went on in his letter, "*exactly* (with exact formulae etc.) how brain material should be prepared for such a study." When Zigas had sent a brain to Melbourne earlier, it was not prepared properly for scientists to study it intensively. Gajdusek wanted to do better.

In mid-May, Gajdusek had his chance. A little girl had died and her mother agreed to an autopsy in return for axes, salt, and a *lap-lap* (a large handwoven bag). Gajdusek did the autopsy in secret, in a hut, at two in the morning, by the light of a kerosene lamp as driving rain and a fierce wind raged outside. The only tool he had to remove the brain was a carving knife, which meant that the brain was mangled as it came out. Gajdusek removed the girl's organs too. If the organs were diseased, that could give hints about the sort of disease he was dealing with: a poison, for example, might ravage the liver and then travel to the brain. But the girl's organs looked normal to him and the only thing wrong with the brain that Gajdusek, who was not trained as a neuropathologist, could decipher was that its hard coating, the dura, looked thick.

"We got the 'dastardly deed' done without awakening much local curiosity or attracting too much attention to our butchery," he wrote in a letter to colleagues. He sent the brain to Melbourne.

He ordered an autopsy knife from Melbourne as well, and the next time he performed an autopsy, he was able to remove the brain in good enough shape for a thorough exam. Gajdusek once again sent it on to the experts in Melbourne. The brain was full of holes, they reported back, like a sponge. Gajdusek sent another brain. It had the same unusual appearance. If kuru was an infection, it was like no infection they had seen before.

By July, Gajdusek and Zigas had met 150 kuru patients and had more than a thousand file cards detailing their clinical history. It enabled them to establish an epidemiology of kuru. Those files, Gajdusek boasted, "represent hundreds of miles of walking and climbing in rugged New Guinea mountains."

There was enough information for Gajdusek and Zigas to write a paper describing kuru, chronicling the blind alleys they'd ventured down trying to understand the disease. They submitted their manuscript to the *New England Journal of Medicine*. Gajdusek entreated his mentor and patron, Joe Smadel, to use his influence to get the paper published.

"Joe," he wrote, "please urge the *NEJM* to get our paper out. . . . They have a chance at the 'first report,' and I think it is worth taking!!" A month later, he wrote to Smadel again: "Please, should you hear from the *NEJM*, assure them that kuru is no figment of my imagination but is a really exciting disease of great importance, for I am sure that is the case."

Their paper was accepted; it would appear in the November 14, 1957, issue of *NEJM*—eight months after Gajdusek had arrived in New Guinea. It described the disease in the patients Gajdusek and Zigas were following and their efforts to zero in on a cause. The disease pattern made it look like kuru was an infection, but every test for an infection had come up negative. But they also could not find a toxin. Nor could they find a clear genetic pattern of inheritance.

Gajdusek still believed that he might find answers in the brains of the Fore. He sent one brain of a fifty-year-old woman with kuru to a neuropathologist at the NIH, Igor Klatzo. Like the previous brain, this one too was shot full of microscopic holes.

In addition, the myelin, a fatty substance that wraps around nerves, insulating them, was ragged and thinner than normal in some places and missing entirely in others. Gajdusek sent more brains. Half of them had rough Brillo-like areas—amyloid plaques. A German doctor, Alois Alzheimer, had seen plaques like that at the turn of the twentieth century in patients with the disease that came to bear his name. To date, they were unique to that brain disease. But children did not get Alzheimer's. And children with kuru had plaques as well.

Klatzo sent his thoughts, along with his report, to Gajdusek about the cause of the abnormalities after examining seven brains. "The closest condition I can think of is one described by Jakob and Creutzfeldt," he explained in his letter dated September 15, 1957. It was a rare disease, abbreviated CJD, and unknown to most doctors. CJD had not been known to affect children, but the resemblance was too close to ignore. There were similar brain lesions but also a similar clinical picture, with trembling and loss of muscular control.

CJD had first been described in 1920 by a German doctor, Hans Gerhard Creutzfeldt, who published a report on "a new and unusual type of neurological disease" he'd seen in a twenty-two-year-old woman. Her illness had progressed in much the same way as kuru in the Fore: starting with tremors and an unsteady gait, moving on to involuntary eye movements, jerking limbs, and dementia. She died a year after the disease began. The next year, another German doctor, Alfons Maria Jakob, had reported four more patients with similar symptoms. The brains of CJD patients had lost nerve cells and had a characteristic spongelike appearance, the doctors wrote.

But by December 1957, Gajdusek contemplated defeat. None of his hypotheses had even a shred of evidence to support them. There could be a link to CJD—Klatzo was a brilliant scientist and it was hard to dismiss his observations—but all he had suggested was that the brains *reminded* him of CJD brains. It was not possible to prove that they were CJD brains.

In desperation, Gajdusek circled back to the idea that the disease was caused by a microbe, an infection. He wrote to Edward Graeme Robertson, a pathologist at the University of Melbourne who had examined some of the brains. Even though Robertson had found no evidence of a sudden or chronic infection in kuru victims, Gajdusek wrote, at this point there was nothing else left to investigate. He knew that infection was unlikely but "kuru is a highly 'unlikely' disease," wrote Gajdusek, and so he wanted to return to this "wild possibility."

All along, as he'd studied kuru, Gajdusek had photographed healthy Fore and kuru victims, publishing photos in the *New England Journal of Medicine* and other medical journals. Soon television crews began to arrive, asking to film him and the Fore. He rehearsed the various potential causes. His references to a cannibalism connection among a Stone Age people proved irresistible to the media. Within a year, he had become something of a celebrity in Australia, the United States, and other developed countries. But still Gajdusek had no answers.

He returned to the United States for a visit, where the cutting-edge labs at the National Institutes of Health offered him a chance to look again for evidence of an infection. The plan was to try to transmit kuru from blood or tissues of patients to laboratory animals. But again he was stymied. The animals remained healthy.

Where Gajdusek's hard work failed, however, his fame offered an opportunity. He received a letter from an American veterinarian, William Hadlow, who happened to be doing research in England on scrapie, a peculiar disease afflicting sheep. Its name referred to the way infected sheep behaved—they scraped themselves raw against fences. Veterinarians had spent decades studying scrapie and were nearly as puzzled by it as Gajdusek was by kuru. But they did have one clue: the sheep could transmit the disease from one animal to another just as an infection would travel, although the doctors could not isolate the infectious microbe.

At the suggestion of a friend, Hadlow had visited a traveling exhibit curated by Gajdusek as part of his publicity push on the Fore. Amazingly, the slides of kuru brains and the descriptions of their victims' symptoms were identical to those of sheep with scrapie. In both diseases there was massive brain cell death, loss of myelin, and—tellingly—the same spongelike appearance that veterinarians called "soap-bubble holes."

In addition to describing the similarities in the letter to Gajdusek, Hadlow published his observations in *The Lancet,* a prominent British medical journal. His conclusion: "I do not suggest that these diseases are identical or even counterparts. But in my opinion their overall resemblance is too impressive to be ignored."

Hadlow also revealed in his letter to Gajdusek that veterinarians could give scrapie to a healthy sheep by injecting the animal with brain cells from another that was sick with the disease. The trick with scrapie, Hadlow wrote, was to wait a long time for symptoms to emerge after that injection. Hadlow called the thus far undetectable scrapie agent a "slow virus." The disease could only be transmitted to other sheep or to goats, which are closely related to sheep. So, Hadlow suggested, the best animals for kuru transmission experiments would be primates.

Gajdusek, who had never heard of scrapie, began to obsessively study the literature. Hadlow was right: the diseases followed similar courses and had many of the same symptoms—problems walking, tremors, changes in behavior. They both ended fatally, usually within six months. And the brains of the victims of both diseases bore soap-bubble holes.

Suddenly, Gajdusek had a renewed zeal for the infectious disease hypothesis. He would use monkeys or chimpanzees instead of mice, following Hadlow's advice, and allow a substantial amount of time for the disease to unfold. It took a while to set up a primate colony under the auspices of the NIH, but finally, on September 17, 1963, one of Gajdusek's close colleagues, Joe Gibbs, working at the NIH lab in Maryland, near Washington, DC, anesthetized and inoculated a chimpanzee with brain tissue from a Fore child who'd died of kuru. And, nearly two years later, a lab technician observed the chimpanzee trembling and falling.

Gibbs sent a telegram to Gajdusek, who by then had returned to New Guinea. Gajdusek flew back immediately to witness the animal's progression. By August, the animal was immobile, unable to survive without constant care. The researchers euthanized her shortly afterward. An autopsy showed that the brain had all the hallmarks of kuru, including the plaques and the holes.

It was settled. Kuru could be transmitted, though, as with scrapie, the agent remained a mystery. Gajdusek settled on using Hadlow's term, "slow virus," even though no one had actually isolated a virus.

Now that he knew a human neurological disease could be spread by this so-called slow virus, Gajdusek leapt at new opportunities. What other human diseases might be transmitted this way? Given Klatzo's observation that kuru brains looked like the brains of patients with CJD, he tried to transmit CJD to monkeys in the same way he transmitted kuru. Further experiments showed that this was indeed possible. What about other diseases? Maybe degenerative brain diseases whose causes were also mysteries—Alzheimer's, Parkinson's, Huntington's, multiple sclerosis, amyotrophic lateral sclerosis, or ALS—were caused by slow viruses? Maybe even chronic illnesses that did not involve the brain, like lupus and Crohn's disease, rheumatoid arthritis, and type 1 diabetes, would fall under the slow virus umbrella.

If he was right, the kuru discovery could transform medicine. It might lead to the discovery of viruses that could be treated. Diseases thought to be random and uncontrollable might be prevented. Gajdusek's mind raced with possibility and ambition. But his hundreds of attempts to transmit Alzheimer's, ALS, and other such illnesses to monkeys failed.

Still, Gajdusek had made the major discovery he had sought. He had proved conclusively that some human degenerative brain diseases—specifically, kuru and CJD—were caused by an infectious agent and could be transmitted. The infectious agent, although termed a slow virus, was unlike anything ever seen in medicine. The brain diseases it caused had none of the hallmarks of any infection that had been studied before. And the incubation period was almost inconceivably long. Gajdusek had discovered a totally new kind of human neurological disease.

As he continued to publish papers and lecture to scientific audiences, his fame continued to grow, as did his public acclaim. In 1976, Gajdusek was awarded a Nobel Prize for his work on kuru.

Given his success and discoveries based on transmitting kuru and CJD to primates—not to mention the primate colony he had developed to allow him to perform such transmission studies—doctors began to send him brains of people suspected of having CJD to confirm the diagnosis.

But another five years passed before Gajdusek stumbled upon the next major discovery. An Australian neuropathologist, ginger-haired Colin Masters, had just arrived to work with Gajdusek at his lab at the National Institutes of Health. Masters's job was to examine the brains that doctors were sending to Gajdusek's lab to be analyzed for CJD. In so doing, Masters discovered that many of these patients had been misdiagnosed and actually had more common diseases like Alzheimer's.

But four of the brains were outliers. They had accumulations of amyloid, the rough hard clumps that are a hallmark of Alzheimer's and can also be seen in kuru. But the plaque in these brains did not look like those in the brains of patients with Alzheimer's *or* kuru. The pathology was somewhere between that of CJD and Alzheimer's. There were too few plaques for Alzheimer's and too many for CJD. And the plaques lacked the distinguishing features of both. When Masters looked at the patients' clinical history, he discovered that each had family members who had died of a similar disease.

Masters recalled a disease he had read about in a paper published in an obscure journal decades earlier, in 1928. Entitled "A Peculiar Heredofamilial Disease of the Central Nervous System: A Contribution to the Problem of Premature Local Aging," the paper described the pathology of a disease that is now known as Gerstmann-Sträussler-Scheinker disease, or GSS.

The author of that paper was a Viennese doctor named Josef Gerstmann. Gerstmann presented the case of a twenty-six-year-old Austrian woman, Berta H., who had an illness that was causing an odd neurological reflex. When the doctor asked Berta to hold her arms out straight in front of her and then turn her head, her arms spontaneously crossed each other so that her left arm pointed to the right and her right arm to the left. She stumbled and lost her balance when she tried to walk. As her disease progressed, she could not control her movements, her speech became slurred, she was irritable, she had a tremor, and her muscles grew weak and flaccid. Soon she could not control the muscles of her tongue or neck; she could not look up at the ceiling.

Later, in 1936, after Berta H. died, Gerstmann and two other neurologists, Ernst Sträussler and Isaac Scheinker, wrote a paper further describing the disease. Berta began showing symptoms when she was twenty-five years old, the doctors wrote, and within a year, was unable to think or reason; she was demented like someone with end-stage Alzheimer's disease. She died six years after the disease had begun, at age thirty-one.

On autopsy, the doctors reported that the dentate nuclei in the woman's brain had degenerated. These are neurons in the cerebellum, the brain region that controls movement. She'd lost myelin, a fatty sheath around neurons that insulates them so that signals can pass among them without interference. The doctors also saw strange-looking plaque—"peculiar inclusions of foreign substances," they described it. Their shapes were distinctive—round or irregular, sometimes with jagged edges. They would mass together in balls or clumps. "These formations are shapes that are rarely found among senile plaque forms," the three doctors observed, referring to plaque found in Alzheimer's disease. In addition, there were holes in the woman's cerebral cortex, the outer portion of the gray matter of the brain.

Gerstmann, Sträussler, and Scheinker also noted that seven other members of Berta H.'s family had suffered the same brain disorder. More than twenty years later, after four additional members of the family had died of what looked like GSS, other doctors calculated the average age of death was forty-six, the disease lasted an average of six years, and that symptoms often included dementia. Eventually, researchers traced the original family's illness back nine generations, starting in the eighteenth century, and reported that at least twenty members of the family definitely had GSS. It seemed to be inherited, and if a parent had GSS, each child had a 50 percent chance of getting it too.

Over the years, doctors from around the world described a small number of families with the same unusual disease: it afflicts fewer than two hundred thousand people in the United States. People would lose their muscle movements, grow clumsy, develop an unsteady gait, and eventually lose the ability to walk and to speak clearly or swallow without choking. GSS remained a rare inherited disorder in the annals of medicine—a medical curiosity with no definitive explanation.

Gajdusek, like most neurologists, knew almost nothing about GSS. But once Masters made that connection, he immediately performed his go-to experiment, trying to transmit the illness to monkeys using brains from GSS patients. He discovered he had found yet another slow-virus brain disease. But it was puzzling.

GSS seemed to be inherited because it only occurred in people related to others who had it—a parent, for example, or a sister. Infectious diseases such as kuru would not spread in such a way. While CJD was also often inherited, showing up in generation after generation of afflicted families in the same way as GSS, it too sometimes cropped up at random in a person who had no contacts with other CJD patients and no family history of the disease. It was hard to see how one slow virus could explain all the variations.

And, most curious of all, even though the infectious agent was being called a virus, it had resisted all attempts to isolate it. That raised questions about what the agent was—and why Gajdusek and his colleagues could transmit GSS and CJD to monkeys; yet at the same time, these ailments were also inherited diseases and, in the case of GSS, seemed to be *only* inherited.

# A Disease

As Gajdusek struggled to resolve these conundrums, unbeknown to him, a young and very ambitious scientist was on his trail. Stanley Prusiner would not rest until he had claimed these diseases for his own.

# 3

# Revelation

Tim had always felt his life was shaped—or perhaps something more like overshadowed—by his exemplary older brothers Billy, Buddy, and Mike. Each had been a stellar student, an honor society member. Each was popular and handsome. Their parents had high expectations for all of their sons and kept them under a tight rein: Buddy later told his wife that leaving for college felt like being let out of prison. Growing up, the brothers bonded in quiet resistance, wrestling in the basement in utter silence so Merle would not come to the top of the steps and ask what was going on; they were always slightly pushing the limits, testing what minor infractions they could get away with without alerting their parents.

In the end, Billy, Buddy, and Mike fulfilled their parents' expectations, growing up to be a dentist, a doctor, and a lawyer, respectively—about as prestigious a group of professions as one could imagine. Only Tim had resisted the pressure to excel. If each of his brothers was going to strive in school, to be at the center of attention, at the top of his class and then his career, Tim decided to take on an opposite role. It was his way of rebelling, assuming what a psychologist once told him was a "negative identity." He did not try to be an exemplary student or an athlete or anything special. He wanted to seem laid back, like someone who didn't care about what was expected of a Baxley. He was the dude who delivered medicines for a local drugstore, driving the business car, a yellow Pinto. He got the job when he was fifteen, the same year he got his driver's license, and kept it throughout high school and through his first year of college. In a continuing effort at rebellion, Tim decided to become a chiropractor after college, a route that won no praise from Buddy, ten years his senior and already established as Hartsville's beloved family doctor. Buddy even asked a revered surgeon in town, Pickens Moyd, to try to dissuade Tim from what Buddy thought was a ridiculous career— to no avail.

Tim's parents, though, were happy to see him find direction, even if it wasn't one they would have chosen for him. They read up on chiropractic practices and did not disparage him.

So Tim got his degree and began practicing chiropractic, enjoying his profession and the close contact he had with his patients. But then, one spring day in 1987, before Bill became ill, when the family was gathered at the family house after church, Tim was struck by a revelation, one that overtook him in a way that he still cannot explain.

Buddy had challenged Tim to a run. They often got into scrappy competitions, even as grown men, still jockeying for position. The two brothers sped along the neighborhood streets lined with tall laurel oaks and headed for a route around the golf course—Buddy, as always, a bit ahead—when suddenly Tim realized something with such certainty, such conviction, that it felt like a blow. It was as though he were being given an order: he was going to go to medical school and he was going to become a neurologist. He'd never before thought about becoming a medical doctor, let alone a neurologist. Yet he now knew that it was his destiny. Nothing like that had ever happened to him before and he was both shaken and exhilarated as he continued to run, awestruck, barely noticing the road beneath his feet.

The brothers sprinted to their parents' house, panting with the exertion, then collapsed into hammocks in the backyard, Tim still tingling from his epiphany. Looking up at the sky he addressed his brother, trying to sound casual. "Buddy, I decided right now that I want to go to medical school."

Buddy was silent for a few minutes, then looked at Tim and warned: "Be careful what you wish for."

Was Buddy telling him that he could never get in, or that he would not like being a doctor? Tim, embarrassed by the way he had blurted out his new calling, let the matter drop.

Though he kept it to himself, Tim felt this lightning bolt of a revelation must have been divine intervention.

He quietly began preparing for his new profession, going back to college to take the courses, like organic chemistry and comparative anatomy, he'd skipped as an undergraduate. He enrolled in the same local college, Francis Marion University, that had given him his undergraduate degree, all the while working as a chiropractor. He made up for the time he was away from the office while in class by working on weekends.

Four years later, he was ready to take the grueling entrance exam for medical school and apply. The same doctor, who tried to dissuade him from becoming a chiropractor, Pickens Moyd, now wrote letters and made phone calls on Tim's behalf. To Tim's astonishment, he was accepted at the Medical University of South Carolina. He paid for medical school by working as a chiropractor during his three-month summer break and on school holidays. Nine years after his epiphany, in the summer of 1996, he had his MD.

Now Tim and Buddy were both doctors. The two brothers would regularly visit each other—Tim was doing his residency training in Charleston, while Buddy remained in Hartsville—

and mull over the mystery of their father's illness, looking for clues, for hypotheses.

All that speculation changed for Tim as soon as he heard that old woman's seemingly offhand comment at his father's viewing in 1998. He knew with a grim certainty that he had to tell Buddy despite the anxiety that instilled in him. Buddy intimidated him. It seemed Buddy still met many of his opinions and theories with skepticism; Tim frequently felt a charge of defensiveness in discussions with his brother. Most crucially, if he told Buddy his fears that their father's disease might be inherited, he would be confronting him with a theory that held a serious family threat within it. He already felt raw from thinking about the consequences if he was right; he didn't look forward to being grilled by Buddy.

The Baxleys were not a demonstrative family, seldom hugging or even touching each other. They had been taught to keep their emotions private, so Tim knew Buddy was unlikely to embrace him in his sorrow and tell him he understood why he was so distraught. No, Buddy might very well just walk away, turning his back on him and his wild imaginings. He had to say something, though. The question was when.

Tim and his family returned to his parents' familiar house after the viewing, weary from the long hours at the funeral home. As soon as they arrived, Tim excused himself, so exhausted he barely made it to the cramped room downstairs where Merle had set up a small bed. It used to be the game room when Tim and his brothers were growing up, where the brothers battled each other in furious games of Ping-Pong. Now it held little more than a couple of narrow beds. But it was still full of mementos preserved by Merle. On shelves lining a yellow cinder-block wall were just about every schoolbook, novel, and nonfiction book her boys had ever owned. Once, Tim's daughter, poking through the shelves, had even found a love note Tim had written but apparently not sent to the prettiest girl in his fourth-grade class; it was carefully penned in his best handwriting on lined paper from his three-ring binder and signed "Love, Tim." And somewhere, tucked away on one of the shelves, was that old World War II compass that symbolized, Tim now suspected, something far more daunting than anyone would have expected.

Next door, in Tim's old bedroom, his wife Janet—tall, kind, chestnut-haired—and their daughters, ten-year-old Parker, Janet's child from a previous marriage, and eleven-month-old Lee, were sleeping. This room was decorated with little more than a painting of a Clemson tiger—all the Baxley boys except Tim had gone to Clemson—and a few pictures from the boys' old yearbooks. All was quiet. Tim envied his slumbering family. His body was exhausted; dead weight, as heavy as if it had been packed with sand. But his mind was alert. It had seized upon the old woman's offhand remark—on its face, so inconsequential—and refused to let go, sending him into a tailspin of visions of the terrifying fates awaiting other members of the Baxley family. He and his brothers tucked into wheelchairs and stationed around Merle's table for Sunday dinner, faces frozen into grotesque masks over steaming plates of food they couldn't even lift their forks to eat. Merle placing flowers on the graves of her husband and sons, tombstones perversely arranged in birth order.

Tim thrashed in his tiny bed, grappling with his thoughts, intermittently reminding himself that he didn't know anything yet. After all, how far could he go with such an offhand remark? So his grandfather had also been a little ungainly—being clumsy doesn't mean anything.

He watched the hours go by. Midnight, 1:00 a.m., 2:00 a.m., 3:00 a.m. He got up and took an Ambien. Four a.m. How would he ever make it through the next day?

He rolled over, a brick of certainty shifting in his stomach. At some point he slept, a heavy dreamless sleep, only to wake again at dawn, dreading his talk with Buddy yet also holding out a slim hope that his brother would convince him his fears were groundless.

Tim dragged himself to the breakfast table. Merle and Janet had made a big pile of pancakes, his daughter Parker's favorite. Mike arrived, driving the short distance from his own house to his childhood home. "He told us at the end that he was just tired," Mike said, struggling with his emotions. "Sometimes death is not the worst thing." Merle agreed. Bill was in a better place now, she said, his suffering was over.

After breakfast the others drifted in, Buddy and his family and Billy with his son and daughter, each of them dressed conservatively in dark colors, somber and sedate, ready for the funeral.

Tim finished his pancakes—the Baxleys always were good eaters, he thought wryly—grabbed his mug of coffee and eased up from his chair. He crossed the kitchen and stepped into the sunroom, the enclosed porch with those windows his father had had such trouble with at Home Depot. Impossible to escape the memories. Restless, Tim drifted back into the dining area and wandered into the hallway leading back to the first-floor bedrooms. It was lined with family photos, so many there was almost no wall left visible. Tim scanned from frame to frame: his parents' wedding fifty years ago; Merle holding Billy, her first baby; the boys going fishing with their dad; Bill and Merle ringed by their entire family at Christmas.

And then there was the photo from Tim's wedding in 1994. Such a bittersweet memory of how things used to be. In it, Merle and Bill and the four Baxley sons with their families stand facing the camera in three lines, the tallest in the back. Ten-year-old Amanda, Buddy's youngest, is in the center of the first row, hands clasped in front of her, shining bangs grazing her eyebrows. Buddy's glasses glint. Bill looks dignified with a white handkerchief peeking out of the breast pocket of his suit. Merle, in a flowered dress pinned with a white corsage, is standing in front of him. It was the last time they were together before Bill's illness accelerated, the last time he could participate in a wedding, the last time of innocence before torment rained down on the family.

Everyone was healthy now, but for how long? If he was right—if the disease was inherited—then they were already running out of time. Tim shook the thought from his mind and looked over at the kitchen where his mother was cleaning up after the meal. She'd been buoyed by the crowd at the viewing the night before; now her years of rigid self-discipline were allowing her to get through this day, at least this part of it.

The long black limousines from the funeral home arrived. It was time to go.

The service was held at the First Baptist Church, a stately redbrick building with four white pillars in front and a stark white steeple against a cloudless blue sky. Bill and Merle had been married in the little chapel behind the church. It was the church where Tim and each of his brothers had been baptized; where they had spent so many Sunday mornings; where their father was a deacon and where he taught a Sunday school class.

Inside, sun streamed through giant stained-glass windows. The mourners continued to file in, filling every pew and packing into the back. The family was among the last to arrive, opening the heavy white doors and seeing the waiting crowd, feeling all eyes on them as they slowly walked down the aisle to the first pew. Bill's casket, closed now, was positioned in front of the pulpit. Bill's only siblings, Faye, who lived in Huntsville, Alabama, and Burt, who lived in Los Angeles, walked in with them. No one had seen Burt or Faye for years. They lived far away and the Baxleys were generally not ones for staying in close touch with relatives beyond the immediate family. So Bill and his siblings had drifted apart. But when Mike, with his genteel ways, always the brother to deliver bad news, had called to say Bill had died, they came.

The minister, Charles Roberts, was an old friend of Bill's, a slender man with a broad ruddy face, a goatee, and bifocals perched on his nose. Despite their thirty-year difference in age, the two would play golf and go to the men's club at church together. Charles recalled his dear friend Bill, told a few stories, described his great character, and then closed on a wistful note: "We will meet again on that beautiful shore."

After the final prayer, the minister looked at the casket and said, "I love you, Mr. Bill."

The family, faces tracked with tears, made their way slowly down the aisle as the organ played a final hymn. Tim escorted Merle, her exhaustion and sorrow weighing her down once again. He slipped his arm in hers, her fragile hand gripping his bent arm as if it were a crutch. They made their way behind the church for the graveside ceremony, a private moment for the family alone. As they slowly walked past the chapel to the little cemetery, Merle looked up at Tim and, with an expression of utter sadness, remarked, "We are right back where we started."

It took Tim a few minutes to understand what she meant—that this was where her life with Bill had started, fifty years before. Their life together was ending where it had begun. Tim stopped with his mother under the shade of some oak trees, hoping for some respite from the intense heat of the day, watching the casket make its slow, measured descent into the freshly dug grave. Bill and Merle had purchased the family plot years ago—there were places reserved for Tim and his brothers too. The fact that his body would one day occupy this ground had always struck him as a detail from someone else's life. But now the reality of his uncertain fate gripped him. His mother crumpled at his side in sorrow; he couldn't imagine putting her through this again. He needed to find answers.

Afterward, the family and a crowd of about sixty friends gathered at Merle's house. In a blanket effort at consolation, everyone had brought food. There was fried chicken. There was basket upon basket of biscuits as well as cakes, potato salad, macaroni and cheese. Merle set it all out in the kitchen, spread it over every surface she had. Her little house—a 1960s-style brick ranch with a living room and dining area separated from the kitchen by a single counter—was once again full, people hurrying back and forth to fill plates and pour cold sweet tea. There would never be alcohol in her home—she had seen firsthand how alcoholism can ravage families and lead to early and tragic deaths. In reaction, she had never touched a drop. She did not even use vanilla extract when she baked because it contained alcohol.

Faye and Burt sat in the sunroom on the other side of the kitchen. Mike saw them there and remembered, as Tim had earlier, the day his father could not figure out how to get the windows into his station wagon.

It had been such a painful time, Mike recalled, those years of watching his father struggle, watching his mother veer between exasperation and pity. It had not been easy to live with Bill after he got sick. Even when he was still able to lurch around the house, still able to shower and dress himself, everything took so long. Merle struggled to remain patient even as she felt such shame to be tired of life with her struggling husband. By the time Bill died, Merle had begun to wonder if she'd have to send him to a nursing home, something she had sworn she would never do. But here, now, as her house filled with people, Merle responded with her usual grace; her sons noticed the way she was strengthened by this outpouring of love and support.

Meanwhile, Tim had been trying to choose the right moment to speak with Buddy, practicing how he would articulate his concern to his big brother. With so many people in the house, with the din of everyone's conversations, Tim realized the time had come: nobody would notice if the brothers disappeared for a few minutes.

He sidled up to Buddy. "Can we talk privately for a minute?" Buddy nodded and the two brothers padded down the narrow hall, past the gallery of oblivious family members and toward the master bedroom, a preferred spot for secret conferences.

Tim's throat was dry as he turned to face Buddy. How to phrase it so as not to sound paranoid? But Buddy seemed ready to listen, leaning against their parents' gleaming dark cherry wood bureau. Tim inhaled deeply and charged ahead. He moved systematically through the chain of events, explaining how he knew it might sound crazy but he just had this feeling about what it meant; how the elderly woman's story had sent goose bumps prickling up and down his limbs and his stomach had dropped under the weight of his intuition. "Maybe it isn't much," he concluded, "but we can't afford to overlook any detail."

Buddy was silent for a few moments. He looked directly at Tim, locking eyes. "You're not wrong," he agreed. "We're in no position to discount a clue, however small." Everything they tried—and they felt as if they had truly tried everything—had ended at a brick wall. They needed a new direction. And if Tim was right—if their father's mystery disease was a thing that could be transferred from father to son and if it could kill you at fifty like it killed their grandfather—well, fifty wasn't far off.

A wave of relief washed over Tim. He was no longer in it

alone. "What about getting that spinal fluid tested?" he asked hurriedly—referring to the fluid they'd drawn from their father and stored in Buddy's freezer. Tim had considered that option when he'd tossed and turned with this news on his own the night before. When they'd first stored the fluid he had no idea what to look for in it, but Tim now knew there was a protein, called 14-3-3, that was nonspecific but if it was present in their father's fluid, Tim explained, it would mean Bill had had a neurodegenerative disease. His symptoms certainly were those of such a disease.

Buddy looked down. "I guess I never told you," he confessed. "We had a power failure a few weeks ago and everything in the freezer thawed. I had to throw out the spinal fluid."

"You've got to be kidding me," Tim replied. At this point he had come to expect disappointments, but this was incredible. Still, what could he say? The fluid was ruined. Anger was not going to solve the problem. It was one more difficulty in what seemed to be a series of unyielding challenges.

The brothers stood staring at each other in the sunny bedroom, the mystery threatening to overcome them, until they were struck with this idea: the question they needed to answer did not require a medical test. What they really needed to know was whether it was possible to inherit their father's illness. Framing the question this way offered a path forward. They needed a family tree of disease. They needed to find every relative they could, tracking down cousins, aunts and uncles, great-aunts and great-uncles, going back through the generations to find out if anyone else had had a disease like the one that killed their father and, perhaps, their grandfather.

But neither brother wanted to take on the project. It would take so much time to find and call long-lost relatives. Both of them had demanding jobs and families. And those calls would not be easy to make, considering the underlying message.

"Mike can do it," Tim decided. Mike was not married. He was the politician in the family—he had just finished twelve years as a state congressman and he knew everyone in the area. He could put anyone at ease.

They'd take Mike aside the next Sunday, when they all went to Merle's for dinner after church, the brothers decided. For the time being they would keep their other brother, Billy, out of it. They felt a slight distance from Billy growing up, despite all the games and pranks they'd played together. Billy tended to keep to himself when his brothers played wild games of basketball in the driveway and begged off their hunting and fishing trips.

Now he lived across the state, working as a dentist in Abbeville. He was going through a divorce and having a difficult time. No, Buddy and Tim decided, asking him was out of the question.

The two brothers emerged from Merle's bedroom, discreetly closing the door behind them. They rejoined the family, keeping mum about what had transpired.

# 4

# An Uncertain Inheritance

At Merle's house the next Sunday, once Merle had served dessert and the meal had ended, Buddy looked at Tim meaningfully. The brothers took Mike aside, bringing him into the master bedroom where Tim and Buddy had convened the week before. Tim explained what the woman had said to him about their grandfather, feeling a bit calmer with Buddy at his side. He spoke of his terrible premonition that it meant this was not the last they'd seen of this illness.

Mike looked at his brothers, trying not to let his astonishment show. He had not intended to keep it a secret, but actually, he already knew about his grandfather's stumbling.

One afternoon, when Mike and Bill had been playing golf, Bill began talking about his father and his work. Then, ever so casually, Bill remarked that men who worked at the mill with him were shaken by what they saw. "They remembered him stumbling from side to side in the textile mill. When you stumble in a mill, a machine can snatch you in. There are a lot of folks around here who are missing fingers and limbs that they gave to the textile mill."

Yet, it had never occurred to Mike to link his grandfather's problem to his father's disease. The main thing that struck Mike was that even though Bill had not seen his father's stumbling and lurching for himself—he'd been away fighting in World War II throughout his father's entire illness—he had heard that people in the factory had been afraid for his father.

Now Mike was astonished that he had missed the connection. And he also realized that if Bill had connected his own symptoms to those of his father, he'd kept it to himself.

Mike agreed that a family tree was a good idea—but even as he agreed to do it, he felt daunted at the prospect. If distant relatives had not known about this disease, who was he to inflict that knowledge on them? Before he began, he wanted to investigate further if his grandfather and his father might have had the same illness.

Tim and Buddy suggested Mike start with Bill's younger brother, Burt, out in California, to see what he remembered. They hadn't seen Burt in years, until the funeral, had rarely even talked to him on the phone. They also considered Bill's sister, Faye—five years younger than Burt, ten years younger than Bill—but she had Parkinson's disease, with its characteristic trembling and shaky voice, making it difficult for her to speak and hard for her to be understood. No, Burt was a better bet.

Burt had an adopted son, Dean, but that meant that if the disease had been passed on to Burt by some horrible chance, if Burt was starting to show symptoms, the disease would stop there.

When Burt answered the phone, Mike saw him again in his mind's eye—he was heavier than Bill, but his eyes, his hair, and his full lips were all Baxley.

Mike remembered Burt sitting in his mother's house the day of the funeral. The funeral. His dad. The pain was still so raw. His voice thick, he explained to Burt what the situation was. Then, forcing himself not to let tears choke him, Mike posed his question. "Do you remember anything unusual about the way your father died?" Burt struggled, trying to dredge up details. Finally, he thought of one that stood out. Bill's and his father, William H. Baxley, Mike's grandfather, had died curled up on the couch in "kind of a fetal position," Burt recalled in an offhand manner.

Mike mulled over this remark for hours after they hung up, flipping and turning it around, as if examining one puzzle piece in a pile of hundreds he couldn't fit together yet. It seemed like a strange posture, possibly significant. It wasn't much, but it was better than nothing.

The next day, dropping in on Buddy in his office in town, Mike repeated what Burt had told him. Buddy was silent, looking at Mike as he considered what to say. Then, weighing his words, he offered his opinion. That sort of detail may not really mean much, but, he told Mike, it probably meant their grandfather had not died of a heart attack or an illness like pneumonia. You don't curl up and die under those conditions. Neither do you curl up and die with a brain disease like Parkinson's. Mike had come away with a clue. Whatever the disease was, it did not seem like something familiar.

Mike knew he had to continue with this project, difficult as it seemed. He would start by working through the few relatives he knew and fanning out to the branches from there. Best-case scenario, the branches would be free of disease, nothing unusual in anyone except his father and grandfather, who may not even have had the same thing. But he also might establish the transmission of disease through generations of Baxleys, retracing their genetic steps to pinpoint the moment the fate of the family was sealed. At least it would be an answer.

Buddy's wife Kathy had offered encouragement in the form of a birthday gift—a computer program to build a family tree. Mike took the floppy disk to his law office that Sunday night. The place was quiet; it was a three-man firm and his partners were home with their families. He installed the software, observed how it worked. Then he went home, dreading what lay ahead.

There was one last shred of hope that he would not have to make those calls. The report on Bill's brain autopsy would be coming in soon. Perhaps it would reveal that whatever had killed Bill Baxley was not hereditary.

Mike delayed for a month, waiting for that report. Finally, he got a call from Buddy. He'd received the brain report from the Medical University of South Carolina. Ripping open the envelope, Buddy read what it said, with a growing sense of dejection: "The morphological findings in this brain best support a diagnosis of Alzheimer's disease. The changes in the substantia nigra indicate there may have also been an element of Parkinson's disease. While many diffuse plaques are found and are very numerous in all areas of the cortex there is no evidence of other brain stem system disease."

Buddy showed the report to Tim who, as a neurology resident at MUSC, knew the vice chairman of neurology, David Bachman. "Being a medical resident is kind of like being in the military," Tim told Mike. Bachman was his attending physician, in charge of his tutelage as he learned to care for patients, and, like all of the residents, Tim always deferred to him. He had another tie to Bachman too. When his father was alive, he'd taken him to Bachman, hoping for a clear diagnosis; Bachman, along with everyone else, had been stumped.

So when Tim approached Bachman in his office, it was with an air of polite respect. "My dad passed away under what I believe to be mysterious central nervous system circumstances," he said. "Would you be willing to take a look at his brain?"

"Yes, I'd be glad to," Bachman replied. A couple of days later, Tim borrowed the slides of his father's brain from the pathology lab in the hospital basement and brought them to Bachman.

Bachman slipped the first slide into a microscope with an eyepiece for Tim so he could see too. They stared at the thin slice of Bill Baxley's brain. So strange to look at his father's brain, Tim thought. Almost unholy. And so hard to look at it objectively. There was no doubt that it was abnormal, though—spotted with plaques, stained brown with the dye used to reveal them, looking like moles, dozens of moles, dotting the brain tissue. And there were tangles—twisted, distorted strings of proteins looking like spaghetti in the brain. Both are seen in the brains of people with Alzheimer's disease. Bachman told Tim he agreed with the neuropathologist who had written the report on Bill's brain. That pathology was consistent with Alzheimer's.

Tim tried to politely disagree. His father had nailed the final question on *Jeopardy* just two weeks before he died, Tim said. The family had just finished dinner at his parents' house and they were all watching the game show on television. When it came time for the final question, Bill took a deep breath to laboriously force out a feeble sound—and he'd given the right answer. "Way to go Dad, you nailed it," Tim told his father. Mike, sitting next to him, patted him on the back. A person with advanced Alzheimer's would never have the mental ability to do that. The disease robs people of their memory and reasoning. An Alzheimer's patient would not even remember the game of *Jeopardy* and would forget the questions as soon as they were asked.

"That's very interesting," Bachman responded, but Tim saw that he was not going to reconsider his diagnosis. And Tim, not wanting to argue with the head of his department, let the matter drop.

No one in this family of doctors could accept Bachman's conclusion. Bill's symptoms just did not match those of Alzheimer's. And it wasn't just that *Jeopardy* question. Alzheimer's didn't explain the paralysis. It didn't explain the chronic fatigue. And Bill knew, as far as any of them could tell, who he was and where he was; he'd never seemed disoriented the way an Alzheimer's patient would. People with Alzheimer's are unable to remember things just said; they tend to ask the same question over and over again, forgetting they've asked, forgetting the answer. Bill never did that. And they stop recognizing their family and friends. Bill never forgot that Merle was his wife or that Billy, Buddy, Mike, and Tim were his sons. The only thing Alzheimer's could explain was the mole-like plaques freckling Bill's brain and those twisted tangles—not to be discounted, certainly, but the plaques looked oddly lumpy for Alzheimer's, the tangles too sparse. So they sent Bill's brain to Duke for a second opinion. But the answer was the same: Alzheimer's.

Once the brothers heard this seconded by the doctors at Duke—seemingly offering a diagnosis rather than admit to anything baffling about the case—they more or less gave up on the medical establishment. And Mike knew that he would have to go ahead with his family tree.

He began by making a list, cataloging the relatives who seemed promising leads. He didn't really know his cousins, but his mother did, at least a few of them. It was the name of an acquaintance, however, that proved most helpful—one that came to his mother suddenly one day, out of the blue.

It had been years, after all, since she'd seen Norma Rainwater, a woman who lived in the South Carolina town of Camden, thirty-five miles from Hartsville. Norma had grown up there near a couple of Bill's uncles. Camden was like Hartsville—people knew one another. They paid attention to the details of their neighbors' lives. And they were happy to share these details with people they knew.

Merle found Norma's number in the telephone book and

Mike gave her a call. Mike had come to realize that he had to go outside the family to find someone who knew how to find family members who had become so distant.

"We were not strangers to Norma—we just had not seen her in years," Mike reminded his brothers, reporting on his progress. "She turned out to be a fount of information. She had, through the years, kept up with everybody and she could tell me about people in our family. From there I just tried to piece things together. Who was who's father and mother. Who the cousins were. Who were the aunts and uncles."

Mike dreaded making those calls. His throat clenched whenever he reached relatives he had never met—who had probably never heard his name—not because it was awkward or embarrassing, but because they might pick up on the implicit implication of his questions: this impending death by slow, painful, and complete deterioration might befall me in the coming years, and by extension, you.

The project posed an impossible ethical dilemma. As much as Mike wanted to know—needed to know—what had happened to his father and what might happen to any of them, he didn't feel it was his right to force that knowledge upon others. His extreme desire to know butted right up against these strangers' right to remain ignorant—it was a matter of life and death for many of them, whether they realized it or not.

Unable to reach an ethical conclusion, he moved forward, continuing his calls. In each case, he did his best to maintain a neutral tone as he gave the reason for his call: "Our dad died recently and I am looking to see whether there are any similar illnesses in the family. Would you tell me please, when your parents died, what was their health status? What was it that your parents died from and what were the symptoms?" He asked about siblings—were they alive, were they healthy, and if not, did anyone know what was wrong with them?

He kept waiting for the angry reply, the phone quickly hung up as the distant relative railed against this stranger with his terrifying call. But it never happened. It was almost eerie. No one seemed to pick up on the underlying message. Or if they did, perhaps they were too polite, or too stunned, to ask probing questions about what Mike was really after.

One of the first relatives he found was a cousin named Harry Stokes. Harry's mother was a Baxley, a sister of Mike's grandfather. Harry had lived in Alabama for thirty-five years and had lost touch with the Baxley family. He told Mike that his mother, Mike's great-aunt, had had what was thought to be a stroke and had died. That was years ago, Harry said, adding that when she died, she had "curled up in a fetal ball."

Mike felt the ground drop out beneath him. His great-aunt and his grandfather had died in exactly the same way. Of course it wasn't quite enough. Mike couldn't quite situate this unusual death posture on the larger spectrum of Baxley family medical oddities. And Bill—who was severely stooped at the end of his life—did not curl up when he died. But it was a strange detail and probably not a coincidence.

The calls continued. Mike learned of more relatives who had died young—of diseases labeled Parkinson's or of seizures or of other mysterious, uncertain causes. He found people with neurological symptoms similar to those his father had exhibited; people who never received a diagnosis.

Mike was beginning to be able to paint a portrait.

It took Mike a year to compile his family tree. The Sunday after it was ready, he brought it to Merle's house for the grand unveiling after the usual post-church meal. His brother Buddy was there with Kathy and their children. Tim and his family came too. Billy, who lived farther away, had not been able to come. (Mike told him later, when he came to Hartsville for a weekend to visit his family.)

After the Baxleys had finished dinner, the kids were dispatched to the game room in the basement. Then Mike peeled back the tablecloth and spread his printout of the Baxley family tree across Merle's heavy maple dining room table. He'd taped four long pieces of white paper together in a smooth line, each family member's name neatly entombed in a tidy box. Mike marked each instance of unusual and untimely death—of dementia, paralysis, seizures—with a small red check: tiny markers of suspicion. He was conservative—"curling up in a ball" was not indicated since he had no idea what symptoms preceded it. But there was enough without it. The diagram plotted, for the first time, a definite trend—a grim inheritance.

The tree had about thirty-five family members in four generations. Mike had put a red check next to Bill and a red check next to two Baxleys in the generation before. He had found one person in the generation before that who seemed to have the disease.

"To me it was just incontrovertible," Mike said. "There was something in our family that was more than just coincidence. There was something in our family that was killing us."

Buddy and Tim warned against jumping to conclusions. How did they really know that those vague disease descriptions, with no medical records, all of which relied on people's memories of events that took place decades ago, were really the same thing? And even if they were, what if everyone in the family who got whatever the disease was had been exposed to a toxin in the environment, some sort of chemical in the air or soil or food, for example?

But even Buddy and Tim did not really believe these alternative hypotheses. For one thing, they didn't all live in the same place, making an environmental toxin unlikely. And the disease's victims had been separated by decades.

The family tree seemed undeniable. This inscrutable disease had been in the Baxley family for five generations.

The Baxleys always felt they were special, but if you'd asked any of them to tell you why, none would have named a medical anomaly as the thing that set them apart. Strength, maybe. Spirituality. Hard work or those bulletproof family values. But never a rare genetic disorder. As mystifying as the disease remained—as directionless as each of them still felt, sitting before a map and having no idea where it would take them—they derived a certain comfort in knowing it existed. In knowing they were not wrong.

And they had a feeling that that family tree might be the start of their salvation.

Mike would look back on that day and tell his mother he saw a message that urged him forward. "The graph was on the table and there was a light kind of shining on it from outside, which is so odd because it was like a graph of death. But there was that shaft of sunlight to tell us there is light, there is hope."

# 5

# Truth like Science Fiction

Gajdusek had been stumped by kuru and the handful of diseases like it. They were infectious, but what was the infectious agent? Calling it a slow virus was what scientists refer to as hand waving: the words sound like they mean something, but when you bear down on them, their meaning evaporates. Slow, yes, but where was the virus?

A scientist named Stanley Prusiner, a neurologist at the University of California in San Francisco, was eager to show Gajdusek up. He'd been working for years on the problem and now, finally, in 1982, he had published the article that described his great discovery. He had found the cause of the strange collection of diseases: kuru, CJD, GSS, scrapie, and a more recently recognized one, fatal familial insomnia, unified by their dramatic and debilitating effects on their victims. It was a major breakthrough by any standard, but Prusiner also knew that what he had found was not going to sit well with his scientific colleagues.

There was no evidence of a virus, Prusiner claimed, slow or otherwise. In fact, there was not even any evidence of an infection: white blood cells were not activated and patients did not seem to develop a fever. So what was this "agent," Prusiner asked, that caused these diseases—that shot people's brains full of holes and yet did not elicit any response from the immune system? He had devoted himself single-mindedly to the project, ceasing to see patients, spending all his time in the lab working with scrapie-infected brains, which were the most plentiful and therefore easiest to get. And he'd come to feel that he owned this problem, thinking of his claim as squatter's rights over what had been Gajdusek's dominion.

Prusiner, like everyone else, had once believed that these diseases were caused by viruses. But he tried six different methods to find a virus and never succeeded.

Then he had a thought that felt almost like apostasy. Could the scrapie agent be a protein? Everything that causes disease—viruses, bacteria, molds, fungi, yeast—contains DNA or its close cousin, RNA. (Genetic information in a cell flows from DNA through RNA to proteins.) DNA is the genetic material; it allows these diseases to reproduce and spread. But everyone knew there is no such thing as a protein that, by itself, with no DNA or RNA around, can cause a disease, or so it was believed at that time. The idea of a protein that somehow reproduces itself seemed like asserting that a cup of egg whites—pure protein—on the kitchen counter could somehow start growing and overflowing the cup, taking over the kitchen like slime in a horror movie.

But as Prusiner began experimenting, every result pointed him in the direction of a protein. Most convincing of all was his discovery that enzymes that chew away at proteins were able to destroy whatever it was that made those brains infectious. Destroying proteins made the scrapie agent disappear..

Still, Prusiner could not quite believe his own findings. His conclusions, he thought, were "beginning to resemble science fiction." Yet, time and again, his results were consistent with his unorthodox theory.

So he submitted a paper announcing his discovery to *Science* magazine. *Science* and *Nature* were, at the time (and still are today), the two leading journals for basic research—just about every scientist reads them each week. Getting a paper published by one of them is considered a mark of prestige and a sign the results are credible and important.

The "scrapie agent," Prusiner proclaimed, was unlike any microbe known to science. It was a protein, but an infectious protein. This was new: it was not at all clear how a protein could even *be* infectious; proteins had always been considered to be inert. By the time he sent his paper to *Science*, Prusiner had even picked a name for these infectious proteins. He'd taken to heart advice he'd been given by Frank Westheimer, a Harvard chemist who'd told him, "Your data are telling you that the scrapie agent is different from anything that anybody has ever seen before. When you have a better idea about the agent's composition, you'll need to spend some time thinking of a name for it. The name is very important. If you choose a bad name, someone else will come along and rename it, and if that happens, your contributions to this discovery may become obscured. But if you pick a good name, it will stick."

Prusiner spent hours trying out and discarding names. One day, sitting alone at lunch, eating a tuna sandwich on rye, he hit upon a good one. He wanted the name to somehow include the words *protein*, *infectious*, and *agent*, so he drew a matrix with *infectious* along the *x* axis and *protein* on the *y* axis. He came up with the word *proin*—that sounded limp to him and he didn't like the way it rhymed with *loin*. Wrong image. But then he reversed the *o* and the *i* to get *prion*.

Prion. He loved it. He said it out loud, PREE-on, and loved it even more. He decided that it would stand for "proteinaceous infectious particle"—and he introduced the name and explanation in the article he sent to *Science*. Then he waited. First came the reviews. Ordinarily, *Science* sends papers to two experts to review. For this paper, it sent it to four. As is customary, *Science* forwarded their anonymous comments to Prusiner.

He read them avidly, deciding three were reasonably positive. But the fourth was scathing, three and a half pages of criticism, calling the paper a "mixture of fact, unproven hypotheses, and unconfirmed personal observations." The reviewer added that Prusiner's contention that the scrapie agent consisted of a protein "depends mainly on the author's own, often unpublished and unconfirmed work." Since Prusiner was one of the few in the world pursuing this project—it was too much of a long shot and it took too long to do for most to want to go after it—his work had indeed gone mostly unpublished and unconfirmed. Scientists had to believe him that he had been excruciatingly careful and rigorous.

Even the term *prion* irritated this reviewer, who realized Prusiner was trying to use the name as a kind of brand. The reviewer complained: "The term PRION is capitalized as if it is a registered trademark. It carries unfortunate echoes of the author's name (PRusiner IONs)."

Ultimately, it is up to the journal's editors to decide what weight to give to reviews and, in Prusiner's case, the decision went in his favor. It is hard to know why because journals cloak their decisions in secrecy. But *Science,* like other top journals, strives for publicity and recognition. A paper like Prusiner's would give the journal that. And if it turned out to be wrong? The blame would fall on Prusiner.

But *Science* took nearly a year to publish the paper. Prusiner was convinced this was out of trepidation. The editors, despite their bravado in accepting it, were worried about how his paper would be received.

When the paper finally did come out, on April 9, 1982— just as Bill Baxley was beginning to complain of "burnout" at work, groping for an explanation for his fatigue—the response was fast and furious. Leading scientists in the field lashed out: Prusiner had not actually isolated this infectious protein. He did not know what it looked like. There were holes in his argument. He could not be correct because the claim that proteins were infectious went against all that was known in biology and medicine.

And, again, the label did not escape criticism. One scientist, Dick Johnson, wrote in a commentary that Prusiner's naming the proteins "prions" without having actually seen them was like naming a baby before you know if it is a boy or a girl. He noted that his own parents had named him Dorothy before he was born, quickly changing the name to Dick when they learned he was a boy. A better name for prions, he suggested, might be "dorothies" for "different or other things with another vowel reversal for euphony."

But Gajdusek's group, still laboring away on the same issues, actually thought Prusiner might be on to something. They too had noticed that the scrapie agent seemed to be a protein and had been trying to decide on a name for it. And they too, of course, objected to Prusiner's effort to put a stamp on it prematurely.

Prusiner was stung by the reaction. Scorn. Outrage. Disbelief. The biting comments and prion jokes never died down. (A decade later, John Hardy, an Alzheimer's researcher, says he congratulated Prusiner on engraving the name "prion" in medical history. Then he added that if he ever found a particle that caused Alzheimer's disease, he would call it a "hardon.")

But Prusiner was not deterred. He went on to propose that the mysterious brain plaques in Alzheimer's disease might be caused by prions as well, theorizing that perhaps the mysterious scrapie agent—the protein that caused prion diseases—was amyloid.

He published a paper in the journal *Cell* in December 1983 laying out this hypothesis. Prusiner gave interviews to the media, pushing the astonishing connection he thought he'd found. "The implications of the findings may be enormous," he bragged to *New York Times* reporter Lawrence K. Altman, before going on to say that prions might hold the key to finding a treatment for Alzheimer's disease.

But even one of Prusiner's coauthors on this study expressed doubts about taking such a leap of faith. George G. Glenner, an Alzheimer's researcher at the University of California at San Diego, told Altman, who quoted him as well in his *Times* article, that he "would be more cautious about the implications until further studies were conducted to prove that prions and amyloid were the same. Later, Glenner told *Discover* magazine, "I have the greatest respect for Stan, but he wanted to get it in the press fast," adding, "I do not think it should have been released at all." Glenner further wounded Prusiner on *The Mac-Neil/Lehrer NewsHour*, stating that it was "mind-boggling to draw any conclusions" about Alzheimer's from the experiments.

In fact, there were good scientific reasons to question this link. Masters and Gajdusek would argue that Prusiner was wrong—unlike kuru and GSS and CJD, Alzheimer's could not be transmitted to primates. There was no infectious protein in Alzheimer's disease. At the time that the *Science* article came out, however, the scientific community was not only challenging the Alzheimer's link but Prusiner's basic hypothesis that infectious proteins caused diseases at all. Charles Weissmann, an eminent molecular biologist at the University of Zurich, told Prusiner he was insisting on a theory that made no sense. Prusiner, he complained, had never actually isolated these infectious prion proteins and shown that they could self-replicate in a petri dish. Weissmann told friends he was amused by the way Prusiner kept insisting on his hypothesis. The idea of infectious proteins "ran counter to all of the basic tenets of molecular biology but that did not disturb [Prusiner] because he was an iconoclast—or perhaps because he was not yet familiar with molecular biology," Weissmann chuckled.

Prusiner stubbornly dug in, continuing to elaborate on his theory. Prions were in fact a natural protein that occurred in all brains, he argued. But sometimes prion proteins are mangled and misfolded into grotesque shapes, although he could not explain how. Those distorted proteins were toxic, he said, and when a toxic prion protein so much as touches a normal one, the normal protein also contorts, becoming toxic as well. The result is like a chain reaction of grotesque proteins in the brain. And when these toxic proteins accumulate they destroy the brain, eroding it and filling it with holes, causing diseases like CJD and GSS and scrapie or kuru.

As for what caused this to happen in the first place, Prusiner proposed two mechanisms. One was a mutation in the prion gene, which directs cells to make prion proteins. If the gene were altered by any number of different mutations it would eventually cause prion proteins to misfold, resulting in a brain disease. So anyone who inherited a mutated prion protein eventually would get one of these brain diseases—which one depended on where the mutation was in the prion gene. Of course, at this point neither Prusiner nor anyone else had found a prion gene, but it had to exist, he reasoned, or there would be no way to explain the inheritance of diseases like GSS.

But that didn't quite square with CJD. Though this illness can be transmitted in the form of mad cow disease when a person eats infected beef *and* can be inherited—both of which would be consistent with the prion hypothesis—more often CJD just shows up on its own, spontaneously. Prusiner explained this away by suggesting that perhaps an environmental insult, like a toxin—or simply bad luck—makes some normal prions misfold, setting off the chain reaction that leads to disease.

Many scientists continued to scoff. Where was the evidence?

Then, in 1987, a forty-one-year-old man came to the University of California in Los Angeles, hoping for a diagnosis. The problems that had begun for him two years before presented some of the hallmark characteristics of these brain diseases—he had trouble walking and difficulty controlling movements of his arms and legs and body.

Bruce Miller, a neurologist at the university, examined the man and took his family history. The man's older sister had died of what looked like the same disease—that is, her symptoms had been the same but her doctors had not been able to figure out what was wrong with her. First, they said she had multiple sclerosis, later changing their diagnosis to olivopontocerebellar atrophy—a shrinkage of some areas of the brain. It was the usual story with a mystery disease—give the symptoms the name of a known disease, even if things don't quite add up. After the woman died, however, an autopsy revealed she had had GSS.

Miller knew immediately that if the sister had GSS, the man had it too. He braced himself to explain to the man what this meant—there was no treatment. He would die as his sister had died. Simultaneously, however, Miller thought to contact Prusiner. He knew he had been working on scrapie and CJD. Did he want to explore GSS as well?

Yes, he did. If he could find a prion gene and show it was mutated in GSS he would gain victory.

Prusiner sent a young associate, Karen Hsiao, to Miller's office to collect the man's blood. Hsiao, who possessed a fiery ambition and youthful hubris, had joined Prusiner's lab just one year earlier. She had gotten a PhD in cognitive psychology and then went to medical school and began a neurology residency at the University of California in San Francisco. And though she had never before even held a pipette, much less worked in a molecular biology lab, she dreamed of finding gene mutations that could cause brain diseases.

One spring day in 1985, Hsiao got her opportunity. Prusiner invited some medical students and neurology residents, including Hsiao, to lunch at a little Mexican café. She made sure to sit next to Prusiner. As she nibbled at her burrito, Prusiner began talking to her privately, ignoring the noisy group at the table. He had a paper that was going to be published in April, he said. He had found the elusive prion gene. It was a normal gene, present in all cells, used to produce prions. The prions were not misfolded—they were normal, harmless prions, function unknown.

A prion gene. That could give them a foothold, Hsiao realized. The goal would be to show that people who inherited a prion disease like CJD or GSS make distorted prion proteins directed by those mutated genes. They could also try to show that others in the family who do not get the disease have normal prion genes and make normal prion proteins. That would be the evidence for the prion theory that everyone had been demanding of Prusiner.

Her heart pounding, Hsiao tried to sound calm and professional. "I want to work in your lab," she told Prusiner. Okay, he told her, but she would have to have her own source of research funds. This meant getting a grant.

It took more than a year for Hsiao to prepare her proposal and get the grant. In July 1986, after her grant money came through, she finally began work in Prusiner's lab.

Not long after that, Bruce Miller called. His patient would come into the UCLA hospital and allow Hsiao to take his blood. She flew there immediately and returned to San Francisco with vials of the man's blood. Then she set to work. It would take two years to look for a mutation in the man's prion gene and discover the gene's sequence. Today, that project would take about two days.

Her goal was to compare, side by side, the two copies of the man's prion gene and see if they were identical or if, as she suspected and hoped, the man had a mutation in one of them.

The work was excruciatingly tedious and the process incredibly technical.

Finally she was ready to do the ultimate test, which would reveal a mutation if there was one.

Hsiao began that final experiment in October 1988, just two weeks after her second baby was born. As it proceeded, she rushed back and forth between the lab and her home, where she nursed her baby. Finally, she was done. She stared at what she had found. There it was—a mutation in the prion gene. This meant a mutation might be the cause of GSS.

Still, Hsiao and Prusiner worried that what they had found in this man's prion gene had nothing to do with his disease. Many genetic glitches have no consequences and genes are likely to differ slightly from person to person, with no obvious change in the way they function. The more genes are studied, the more alterations are discovered. These days, these ambiguous alterations even have a name: VUS, variation of unknown significance.

They needed stronger evidence. They needed to show that GSS only occurred when the gene was mutated. That meant finding a large family with GSS and examining the gene in those with the disease and those who were healthy and had lived long enough to be nearly certain they would not ever get GSS.

By coincidence, Tom Bird, a geneticist at the University of Washington, had recently discovered just the family Prusiner and Hsiao needed. Bird's specialty was Alzheimer's disease; he focused on a rare inherited form of the disease that strikes people in middle age or even earlier. So, in 1984, when a twenty-nine-year-old woman called him and said she was a member of a family with inherited early-onset Alzheimer's disease, he was eager to study her and her family. The woman told Bird that her family had been the subjects in a research study twenty years earlier. Another group of scientists had published a paper reporting they'd traced early-onset Alzheimer's back for seven generations in her family. Symptoms usually began when people were in their thirties or forties. But after that paper was published, no one had followed up, the woman explained.

She sent Bird a four-page handwritten letter discussing her family history and providing a detailed family tree showing who was alive and who had died of Alzheimer's disease. She provided names, addresses, and telephone numbers of family members and added that she'd heard that two cousins in Oklahoma were also starting to develop the disease.

Bird and his research groups gathered medical records and any available autopsy materials. They called family members and contacted the cousins in Oklahoma. One man was so ill with the family disease that he wasn't really able to carry on a telephone conversation. His wife took the call and explained that her husband seemed like he had Alzheimer's disease, unable to remember what he had just said or what he had just been asked, confused, forgetting words.

That man died two years later, in 1986, and Bird arranged for his brain to be sent to the University of Washington for an autopsy. He sat down with a neuropathologist, David Nochlin, and began looking at slices of the man's brain. They saw plaques, the hallmarks of Alzheimer's disease, but they looked funny, clumping together. And some of them had several hard little nuggets at their centers instead of just one.

Bird also noted that there were not many tangles, at least not the typical mass of spaghetti-like twisted proteins that are in Alzheimer's brains.

Bird looked up from the microscope and peered at Nochlin. "What do you think?" he asked. "Could this be a prion disease? And if it is, is there a way we prove it?"

They called Colin Masters, the Australian scientist who had worked with Gajdusek; he had become one of the few experts in diagnosing prion diseases from brain slices. He also was one of the few who had antibodies that would attach to prion proteins, revealing their presence. If it was a prion disease, prion proteins would reveal themselves in clumps in those plaques.

"Sure," Masters said to Bird. "Send me the tissue."

In August 1987, he wrote to Bird. He had a diagnosis. The family had GSS.

Bird and Masters published their paper two years later, in 1989, the same year that Mike Baxley completed his family tree of disease. It was also roughly the same time as when Karen Hsiao had discovered the prion gene mutation in Bruce Miller's GSS patient. For the Baxleys, the state of the science was too preliminary to help them. But for Hsiao, her moment had arrived. Bird was happy to collaborate with her. Now she could examine whether the gene mutation predicted GSS. If it did, she would have her evidence that mutations in the prion gene caused the disease.

Bird sent Hsiao DNA from the blood he had collected from the family—eighteen DNA samples in all. Sure enough, she found a mutation in every single person with the disease and none in those who had lived long enough to be certain they had escaped the disease. Now Bird knew he could predict, with a blood test, who in that large family of German extraction was going to get GSS. He knew the mutation and he knew that anyone who had it would get the disease. He had blood from ten or so family members who were at risk of getting GSS and offered to test their blood for the gene mutation. Only one wanted to know. He tested positive for the mutation, and, indeed, he died of GSS at age thirty-nine. (The young woman who'd originally brought her family to the attention of Bird developed GSS but her death, in 1994, was from a brain tumor that Bird believes was unrelated to GSS.) Later, Bird found another large German family with GSS who also turned out to have a prion gene mutation.

For Bird, those discoveries—the mutation in the prion gene and the demonstration that it could cause GSS in two separate families—were proof positive that Prusiner had been right when he said mutations in the prion gene caused the disease.

Bird was impressed. He thought about all the well respected scientists who continued to scoff at Prusiner, but he realized that the prion theory had reached a turning point. All it took was an abnormal prion protein—nothing else—and GSS would emerge. This fact should finally erase any doubts about the relationship between prions and GSS, CJD, scrapie, and kuru.

Meanwhile, Karen Hsiao had inserted a prion gene with the GSS mutation into mice. She was at home when she got the call from an animal caretaker at the lab. One of the mice was showing signs of the disease. The mouse had GSS.

The mouse's misfortune meant that at last they could celebrate. Prusiner surprised Hsiao by giving her a hug—uncharacteristic behavior to say the least. But this was big—now he had yet another strong piece of evidence that he was right about prions. He published this paper in *Nature*.

The skeptics persisted, however, Charles Weissmann among them. It remained possible that a virus caused prion diseases. What if those mutations changed brain cells in such a way that an otherwise innocuous virus could infect them and destroy the brain? After all, the whole prion hypothesis was still based on speculation. No one had isolated abnormal prion proteins and showed that when they touch normal prion proteins a chain reaction occurs.

Then, in 1990, Weissmann thought of an experiment that might settle the matter. Suppose he bred genetically engineered mice that totally lacked the prion gene. That would mean those mice could not make prion proteins. If he injected them with brain extracts from a sick animal, the distorted prion proteins could not cause a chain reaction because there would be no normal prion proteins to react. But if a mouse without prion proteins still got sick after that injection, the prion hypothesis would be basically destroyed. In 1991, he developed the first mice without prion genes. They seemed healthy and had normal life spans. He told Prusiner he wanted to conduct that crucial experiment.

Prusiner was reluctant, telling Weissmann he had other experiments he wanted to do with the mice. He was putting off the moment of truth, Weissmann decided. So Weissmann insisted. A year later, he had his answer. The mice that lacked the prion gene had proven resistant to scrapie. It was just what the prion hypothesis predicted. Since these mice could not make normal prion proteins, the addition of abnormal ones could not set off a chain reaction turning the normal ones abnormal. The mice could not get a prion disease. He called Prusiner. "Stan, everything is working out your way," he conceded.

Gradually, Prusiner and his prion hypothesis gained a grudging acceptance in the scientific community. Even if there were still some diehard skeptics, there was less outright ridicule. In the spring of 1992, he was elected to the prestigious National Academy of Sciences, whose membership is reserved for the most eminent of scientists. He received four awards that year for his research. In 1994, he won a Lasker Award, often said to be a precursor to the Nobel Prize.

For the next few years, friends assured him he was going to get a Nobel. But every October, around noon in Sweden and 6:00 a.m. on the East Coast of the United States, when the prize was announced, Prusiner had to face the fact that it had gone to others. It was worse than just not getting the prize. To him, each year that he did *not* get a call from Stockholm brought with it the unstated assumption that something was wrong with his work. He began imagining spending the next thirty or forty years anxiously awaiting the call from Stockholm. And that call would never come. He worried that the fact that he was passed over every year would vindicate his critics. And he was embarrassed by his naked thirst for the prize. But Prusiner also worried that if he *did* get a Nobel, he would have to share it with Gajdusek, who had written a chapter in a virology textbook claiming he was the first to find the protein causing scrapie. But where, Prusiner asked, were the publications in scientific journals proving Gajdusek's assertions?

In early 1996, Prusiner got a call from Erik Lycke, a friend in Göteborg, Sweden, who had nominated him for a Nobel several times. Members of the Nobel Committee, Lycke confided, "are unclear about Gajdusek's role in the discovery of prions. Gajdusek is telling them that he discovered PrP, which he calls the 'scrapie amyloid protein.'" Lycke suggested Prusiner write him a letter with references documenting the discoveries Prusiner had made.

Prusiner was more than happy to comply. He and Gajdusek had a distant and not particularly cordial relationship. Two big egos battling over one mysterious type of disease. And Prusiner knew that Gajdusek was still a hero for his work on kuru while he himself was still tainted by all those years of ridicule. If

Gajdusek got the prize with Prusiner, all the attention would be on Gajdusek. Prusiner would be reduced to a footnote.

Prusiner imagined the newspaper headlines: "Gajdusek wins second Nobel for his discovery of prions."

But, in April 1996, in a disturbing turn of events, rumors and suspicions about those many boys Gajdusek had taken home to live with him in his Maryland house reached a stunning climax. The FBI, as it turned out, had been investigating Gajdusek for more than a decade. Their interest was piqued by references to his journals—which had been published and distributed by the National Institutes of Health—on child pornography sites on the Internet.

Some anthropologists, reading those journals, also raised concerns. While Gajdusek never directly said he had sex with young boys, he described ritual homosexuality among men and boys in New Guinea villages in ways that veered from standard academic descriptions and that, to some scientists, implied that he was engaging in sexual relations with his subjects. In one instance, he wrote that boys aged six to twelve are the "preferred fellators" of men and then, shortly afterward, a passage declares that he'd experienced a long period of "perfect sensuality and satisfied passion."

In 1996, a twenty-three-year-old college student told the FBI that almost as soon as he arrived at Gajdusek's house from Papua New Guinea, when he was fourteen, the famous scientist had begun sexually abusing him.

The FBI secretly recorded a conversation between the young man and Gajdusek in which the man asked Gajdusek if he knew what a pedophile was.

"I am one," Gajdusek replied.

Still, when Gajdusek was arrested, on April 4, 1996, members of the scientific community were shocked. Three scientists staunchly defended him—even paid his bail, requiring two of them to put up their houses as collateral.

But at his hearing on February 18, 1997, Gajdusek admitted to the charges. He was sentenced to serve up to thirty-five years in prison but ended up with a reduced sentence of one year.

When the hearing was over, Gajdusek turned to one of the scientists who had put up his house to pay his bail and complained bitterly: "You damn dummies didn't even know I was gay."

The day Gajdusek was released from prison he fled to Paris and never returned to the United States. He died a decade later, a broken man.

In 1997, with the Gajdusek threat gone, Prusiner finally got the call from Stockholm. He was attending a conference at the NIH, staying at a Holiday Inn just down the street from the Maryland campus. At 5:00 a.m. the phone rang. Despite all the years he had longed for the prize, he was flabbergasted when he got the news. "For his discovery of Prions," reads Prusiner's Nobel Prize citation, "a new biological principle of infection."

As always, controversy swirled around Prusiner. Critics felt there were still unanswered questions: Yes, mutations in the prion gene can cause diseases, but that does not mean prion proteins themselves are the equivalent of viruses or bacteria. Just because no one has found a virus that causes prion diseases does not mean it does not exist.

But *Science* also reported a defense of the prize by Ralf Pettersson, deputy chair of the Nobel Committee at the Karolinska Institute. "The committee is well aware of where the field stands," Pettersson remarked, adding, "The details have to be solved in the future. But no one can object to the essential role of the prion protein" in these brain diseases.

Regardless, the work had direct implications for families like the Baxleys—although they did not know it yet. Thanks in large part to Prusiner, it was now possible to detect a GSS mutation in the prion gene with a blood test. Which raised the very question that would come to alter the lives of every single member of the Baxley family: Would you want to know if you carried a fatal gene mutation?

# 6

# Birthright

In 1999, three years after Prusiner was awarded the Nobel and just a few months after Mike completed his family tree, the Baxleys began falling like dominoes, one after another succumbing to the mystery disease.

Billy, the oldest brother, the dentist, was first. His early symptoms were innocuous, ambiguous, easy to dismiss. His hand began to hurt while he worked. But he was a dentist, and fixing a person's teeth demands a lot of small movements, meticulous work, or so he reasoned. "It's nothing," he told himself. He must be getting carpal tunnel syndrome.

The next sign did not come until a year later and was harder to hide. Billy had always been athletic and agile and took pride in his balance and strength. He often worked out with his partner, Steve. The two men loved bodybuilding. Billy had gotten so serious about his workouts that he began entering deadlift competitions. He also loved white-water rafting and wanted to tackle every river in the state of North Carolina.

One bright summer day in 2000, Billy and Steve planned a rafting trip on the Oconee River, a wild and challenging waterway that offered the sort of rafting Billy loved. The river wound through mountain forests and featured back-to-back rapids with names like Broken Nose, Tablesaw, and Hell Hole.

His brother Mike came along, as did Billy's son and daughter, seventeen-year-old Davis and twenty-year-old Jennifer. They put on bright yellow life jackets, snapped white helmets on their heads, and climbed into two big, gray rafts. Almost as soon as they hit the river, Billy fell out of the raft, tumbling over the side, plunging into the rushing water. Not long after he got back in, he fell once more. And then again. He couldn't maintain his balance in the pitching raft.

Davis, watching with growing apprehension, tried to excuse the first few falls. Everyone falls on a white-water rafting trip—that's part of the sport. But Billy's falling was excessive. The first few times, Billy pulled himself back onto the raft, only to tumble in the water again. He soon seemed flustered and exhausted, so the others started grabbing his jacket when he fell and hauling him back onto the raft, only to have him fall into the river again. It happened dozens of times in succession. There was a pattern, Davis noticed, and it went like this: Brace yourself. Here it comes. Splash.

Steve was worried too. But he said nothing, just watched as Billy laughed and acted for all the world like he was having a wonderful day rafting.

Jennifer was with Mike in a different raft, behind the others. In that torrent of water, focusing on the pitching raft, she could not see what was happening to her father and did not realize he was lurching out of the boat. But she had seen something troubling earlier. Walking over the river rocks to get into the raft and start the trip, Billy kept slipping and falling. Something is definitely wrong with him, Jennifer thought to herself, worried. They were all having the same reaction, independently, in their own heads, without daring so much as eye contact for confirmation. Jennifer put her concern aside, but it kept coming back. She *knew* that her agile, athletic father should not be slipping and falling on those rocks. That was so unlike him. It frightened her.

That night, Steve broached the subject and Billy confessed that the day had been difficult and that he'd been exhausted trying so hard to stay on the raft. But Billy and Steve kept their worries to themselves, no need to frighten the family just yet. Maybe it was nothing, they told themselves.

After that trip, Jennifer could not get her father out of her thoughts. A few months later, when her uncle Mike was visiting from Hartsville, he and Jennifer went out for dinner. In the middle of their meal, she put her fork down and asked the questions that had been nagging her. "Did you notice anything unusual about Dad when we were whitewater rafting?" she said, then cast her eyes downward. "Did he seem clumsy to you? Do you think something is wrong?"

When she looked back up, Mike looked both startled and concerned. Of course he'd seen it, but he did not know what to say. He was not a doctor. He could not give a diagnosis. Yes, something seemed wrong, but he felt stymied—what would be gained by telling Billy he was unsteady on his feet?

Meanwhile, Davis too was having trouble reconciling that clumsy man who could not stay in the raft with the expert rafter his father had always been. He also struggled with the idea of confronting Billy. His father was quick to anger and it would be such a difficult topic to bring up. There was never the right opportunity.

But a few weeks later, Billy picked up Davis to take his son on a weekend jaunt. As he drove down the highway in his Jeep Wrangler, Billy, looking straight ahead, said, "Hey, on my way home from work today I ran off the road." He did not know how it happened but he had ended up slashing his tire.

"You did *what?*" Davis asked. Billy did not reply. But he seemed scared.

Billy retired later that year, at the age of fifty. His official explanation: he was tired of the hour and a half commute to his dental office; it was a wearying, boring drive. But it was becoming increasingly difficult to deny that the illness had taken hold. The coordination in his hands had deteriorated so markedly that he could no longer muster the strength to pull a tooth. And he'd started experiencing a new and troubling symptom—his arms and hands would suddenly jerk of their own volition. Now there was a real chance that Billy might hurt a patient. And his hands had gotten too weak to write out prescriptions or hold tools. Time was running out on him. He knew he wouldn't be able to work much longer, so he left before the office whispers came to anything substantive.

Over the next few months, Billy's family watched as his motor skills continued to degrade, no one knowing what to say. The changes had, at first, taken place slowly and over a long period of time; it was only after that rafting trip that it became undeniably clear that Billy's vulnerabilities were meaningful. But no one wanted the worst to be true—they didn't want Billy to be next in line after his father. As time wore on, however, it became difficult to imagine it could be anything else.

His brothers had despaired of getting through to him. Billy had made it clear he did not want their pious entreaties, did not want to discuss his lifestyle with Buddy, did not want to hear that his family could not understand him. His brothers felt there was a wall around him that they just could not breach.

One day, visiting at Mike's beach house, Tim watched Billy hobble precariously down the stairs, clutching the railing, summoning all his focus to bend his knees and plot each footstep. The next night, Tim found a private moment with Billy and gently asked him what was going on—if he had considered seeing a doctor; "No, no, no," Billy retorted hotly, "I've got new shoes. It's my shoes." Billy was adamant, but the truth had become brutally obvious. Tim was at a loss. If Billy refused help, what could he do?

The moment of truth for Billy came when he was on vacation with Steve in Key West. The two men had gotten up early to ride bikes before breakfast, but as soon as he mounted his bike Billy began weaving into the road. "Hey," Steve shouted as Billy tried to steer his bike back to the shoulder, only to veer out again. Steve yelled, and Billy steered back to the shoulder only to wobble into the road yet again. "Hey Bill, how about we take a break," Steve said. The two men stopped and got off their bikes. Billy looked at Steve, trying to hide the fear that gripped him. "We haven't even had a cocktail yet," Billy joked. Then he and Steve flung their legs over their bikes, ready to try again. Now things were even worse. Billy could no longer push off with his foot. Riding was impossible. Slowly, shaken by the experience, he and Steve dismounted, turned their bikes around and began walking back to the hotel. Something was wrong, gravely wrong. Back in their room, they embraced in silence. "I have to call Tim," Billy finally said. His brother was a neurologist, He would know what to do.

By that time, after months of silence from his brother, Tim had given up hope of being able to guide Billy to medical attention. He never expected that day when his receptionist burst into his office, at once wary and urgent. "Your brother Billy is on the phone," she announced. Right away, Tim knew something bad had happened. Billy never called him at his office. Knowing that he would be met with bad news, Tim picked up the phone. "I'm on vacation in Key West," Billy said, his voice thick with fear. "I can't ride or even balance on my bike." Tim heard Steve in the background nudging Billy to "tell him about the pushing off part."

"I can't even push off with my foot without falling," Billy added.

Tim took a deep breath and looked down at his desk.

"It will be okay, Billy," he told his brother. "Just come home and my partner Rick will see you. It's going to be okay. We're going to take care of you." But even as he said it, he knew it was an empty promise. After hanging up, Tim sat staring at the wall, stunned. He would have liked to examine Billy—he, after all, knew every detail of their father's disease—but doctors do not ordinarily practice medicine upon their family members. When Tim and Buddy had taken the spinal fluid and skin from their father they were acutely aware of the transgression; Tim did not feel comfortable doing it again. Rick can figure it out, Tim told himself; he would tell Rick what to do. Tim offered a silent prayer. "Please, let this be alcoholism or nitrous oxide abuse—anything but what Dad had."

Rick encountered the bewildering symptoms Tim feared he would and sent Billy to the National Institutes of Health. They agreed to see him—but, as had been the case with his father, even the best doctors could not decide what was wrong. And all the while, Billy's symptoms were worsening, leaving Tim with a sickening feeling of déjà vu every time he saw his brother.

# 7

# Insomnia

Buddy Baxley's dread took hold in the space of a single night. It was April of 2000, the year Billy retired from his dentistry practice. Buddy was forty-eight, busy in his career and happy to be so. He played the role of the small-town family doctor with bottomless enthusiasm. He was the doctor people came to with complaints like sinusitis or a hacking cough. Mothers would bring their babies when they developed a fever or an earache. Amid the parade of these everyday complaints, he spotted the serious cases that needed a specialist's care and was quick to refer his patients when necessary.

He opened himself entirely to the patients who came into his practice, feeding them if they were hungry, caring for them without question if they didn't have the means to pay their bill, and handing out his home number with the sincere instruction to call him anytime, day or night. A man of deep faith, Buddy kept Bibles in his waiting room and bought self-help books by Christian authors, offering them to patients having difficulties—his patients often called him Preacher Doc. He ferried between the clinic and the hospital, keeping watch on his patients in both. Buddy was the only doctor many in Hartsville had ever seen, and his patients loved him for his selflessness and dedication, his gentleness and patience and ability to truly listen.

And he showed his family the same commitment and kindnesses at home. He and his wife, Kathy, a generous woman given to exuberant laughter and animated gestures, had both lived in Hartsville for nearly their entire lives. They'd married when Kathy was just eighteen; Buddy was twenty-four. They had three children: Holly, Luke, and Amanda; the family lived what looked to outsiders like a cliché of complacent small-town life.

For Buddy, life was full and happy. But that night, Buddy lay quietly in bed, watching the slow progress of minutes ticking into hours on his bedside clock, trying to stay still so as not to disturb Kathy lying peacefully beside him. He watched the feeble shaft of sunlight creep into the room as the morning finally came. He felt a stab of tenderness for Kathy—for his slumbering family—as he waited and waited for the sleep he had always taken for granted.

It never came.

The alarm went off at six as usual, but Buddy's eyes were already open. Clicking it off, he lurched upright and swung his feet over the side of the bed, trying and failing to shake the fatigue from his head. He walked into the bathroom and examined his drawn face in the mirror as he shaved—he had the Baxley look, but unlike his brothers, he also had a deep dimple in his chin. Today, his eyes looked heavy, his skin gray. He pulled on his customary khaki pants and slipped a button-down shirt over his slight body, adding a clip-on tie, all purchased at a thrift store whose owner was his patient. Better to just keep mum about his sleepless night, he thought. There was no reason to tell his wife or Amanda, a junior in high school who was by that time their only child still at home. Granted, he was a good sleeper but, really, insomnia was a pretty common problem. It was almost prosaic, the plight of so many of his patients, something he dealt with all the time in others. No cause for alarm.

Then, as he did every day, Buddy got into his 1976 green Ford Bronco and drove to the community hospital. When he arrived, his usual breakfast was waiting for him in the cafeteria, a boiled egg and a muffin. Then he made the rounds, visiting patients in their hospital rooms, praying with those who were going to have surgery or who just needed the comfort of his presence. After that, he drove to his office on West Carolina Avenue, a squat freestanding beige brick building.

He made it through the day. When he finally arrived home, Buddy was so exhausted it felt as if his body were made of lead. Almost dizzy, he lay down to sleep that night, expecting to be out before Kathy switched off the light. But then . . . he found himself counting off the minutes on his clock for a second night in a row. He closed his eyes and tried to breathe slowly and steadily, but his brain only spun into nonsensical thoughts until his alarm drew him from bed again.

The second sleepless night was followed by a third, and a fourth. His days were plagued by an intense dizzying tiredness, his nights by the torture of lying awake. Insomnia became the norm and his life began to unravel.

Even worse, he knew, were the effects on his patients. With no sleep short-term memory can falter: it is hard to concentrate, hard even to pay attention when a patient's health is at stake. For a doctor—who must write prescriptions, make diagnoses, decide whether a patient needs immediate emergency care—insomnia can be disastrous.

Buddy cast around for the cause of his sleeplessness and decided it must be stress over his frustrating dealings with Amanda. His youngest daughter had been an easy child who adored her siblings. When she was little, he had nicknamed her Moon Pie after her favorite snack—later this was shortened to Moon. She'd been her daddy's little Moon since then, his shadow since she'd been able to walk. But after a childhood spent hanging around with her dad, going to his office after school, she changed abruptly in adolescence, becoming more rebellious. Headstrong.

Now Amanda was proving impossible to control. She'd acquired new friends who drank and smoked and seemed to do nothing but seek out trouble—or so Buddy thought. She was the fearless one in her crowd, the one determined to have her way. She and her friends would drive to a gas station that was notorious for selling alcohol to minors. Amanda was always the one who would go in and buy Boone's Farm wine coolers. Her friends made her purchase the drinks because they knew she would, because she didn't care about rules.

Nothing gave Amanda pause and everything her parents discovered about her terrified them. One of Amanda's boyfriends, after drinking heavily, crashed his car into a tree. He survived—but as a quadriplegic. Buddy and Kathy considered what could have happened if Amanda had been with him. Those parties, that drinking. How could they get her to stop?

They tried everything. They would forbid Amanda to talk to a boy. She would hide in a closet with the phone, whispering in the dark. They would take the phone away. She would call from a friend's house. They would deny her request to attend a party. She would climb out of her window and go anyway.

They tried all of the many things that parents have tried for centuries. Talking to Amanda didn't help. Yelling only made her dig in. Buddy's reasoning was not working and neither were the punishments—what was he supposed to do?

Buddy thought about a chilling experience he'd had the day before his first sleepless night. He had gotten together with a friend after work, and the two men began talking over how things were going for them. Inevitably, Buddy brought up his problems with Amanda. He thought his entreaties were finally having an effect. "I think Amanda's coming around," Buddy told his friend.

"No, she's not," Buddy's friend shot back, exasperated. "You have to put your foot down. You are not ruling the roost."

Buddy was infuriated. How much harder could he try to tame his rebellious daughter? At that instant, something strange happened to him. It was like something popped inside his head. That night he could not sleep.

He insisted to himself that it was his difficulties with his daughter that kept him from sleep, pushing aside the knowledge that no matter how much the sea change worried him it wasn't what overtook him at night. In the eternity that opened before him every night, his mind almost never cycled back to Amanda or his patients or any obstacles he'd faced during the day. Instead, he thought only of his inability to sleep, to shut his eyes and surrender to a peaceful night. And now his insomnia was accompanied by something worse, a terrible sense of impending doom.

Every morning, Kathy turned to Buddy in bed and murmured, "Honey, how was it?" Every morning he replied, "It's the same."

"How in the world are you doing the job you are doing when you are not getting any sleep?"

"I don't know. But it scares me."

What was he going to do? Buddy wondered. He could not work if he could not sleep, nor could he maintain much of a family life. He couldn't maintain any kind of life at all. He watched the domestic idyll he'd built disintegrate in his hands, powerless to stop it.

He sought the help of a therapist. He was skeptical of psychotherapy but was now ready to try anything that might help him sleep. The therapist decided Buddy might be suffering from depression and prescribed an antidepressant, Effexor. But Buddy stopped taking it after one day.

"I feel like I am going crazy," Buddy told Kathy as he tossed the bottle of pills into the trash. "I can't control my thoughts. I feel like my mind has gone berserk." And still, he couldn't sleep. At most, he estimated, he drifted off for perhaps two hours of sleep before being jolted awake again.

Buddy remained in this state of involuntary watchfulness— lying awake night after night—for two long years. He told his brothers about his sleeplessness, not wanting to make too much of it. None of them connected it to the family disease—after all, insomnia was not a symptom as far as anyone knew.

# 8

# Naming the Problem

"Oh, by the way, I heard Faye is in the hospital with pneumonia," Merle said in passing to Tim during one of their weekly phone calls. He felt a jolt of fear as he thought about his father's sister. She might have the flu or maybe complications from a bad cold, but Tim had a sinking feeling as he tried to convince himself of this. His heart began to pound as it had when he heard about his grandfather lurching through the factory. As a neurologist, he knew most people with degenerative neurological diseases usually die of pneumonia. His own father had died of pneumonia.

Faye, a scientist at NASA, was divorced and lived alone in an apartment in Huntsville, Alabama. Tim hadn't seen her since his father's funeral. There she'd seemed a bit trembly—but he'd attributed that to the Parkinson's disease he'd heard she had. Tim had not thought to question that diagnosis at the time, even in light of what he'd learned about the family illness. Now he decided he'd better check on her. Merle gave him Faye's number.

He called her and chatted for a bit, not wanting to seem abrupt but also concerned about making her talk for too long because she was obviously finding it difficult to speak. Her voice was strained; her sentences short. She sounded exactly as his father had in his final years. Then Tim finally said it:

"My mom says you haven't been feeling well. It's been a long time since I saw you. Mind if I come by for a visit?"

Faye said she'd be glad to see him. Maybe the peculiar quaver and drag in her voice was nothing but exhaustion or advanced Parkinson's. He resolved to see for himself and blocked out a day to visit Faye.

Before that day arrived, Tim was in his office after hours, his patients and staff gone for the day, because he was on call at the hospital across the street. He sat at his desk, putting these rare idle hours to productive use. He was preparing for his neurology boards; poring over a study guide, his eyes growing heavy under the weight of so many dry case histories. Suddenly, his eye snagged on something that pulled his attention back to the page, holding it there with an uneasy familiarity. The case history involved a young man who had developed ataxia—an inability to coordinate his movements. His brother not only had ataxia but had developed dementia. The diagnosis for these brothers was an extremely rare inherited brain disease: Gerstmann-Sträussler-Scheinker disease, GSS—a lesser-known prion disease in the same vein as CJD, which Tim had studied in school. An expert pathologist can diagnose the disease by examining the brain after a person dies. The idea, which arose from Prusiner's work, is to look for telltale prion proteins by using enzymes to chew up the normal prions in the brain. Then the pathologist floods the brain with antibodies to the misfolded prions that remain. If the misshapen prions are there, the antibodies will glom onto them.

Tim snapped the book closed and began pacing around his small office, weighing the implications in his mind. The mutation that caused GSS was inherited; if you had the gene, you would certainly develop the disease. His father Bill had probably had it; Billy probably had it; Faye probably had it. But then, the disease struck only two to five people out of every hundred million. The chances were so slim—and yet they were real. Those few people—those fifty families in which the disease had been documented—they existed. And they had died from GSS.

Tim rushed home once he was no longer on call at the hospital to tell his wife Janet. What are the chances he would find the name of his family disease, after some of the nation's best doctors had been stumped, simply by studying for his neurology board exam? Perhaps this was the moment that his revelation to become a neurologist during his race with Buddy had been leading to—perhaps this was why he felt so certain when it hit him.

"It was providential," Tim told Janet. "It's as if God wanted to make sure this diagnosis got through my dense skull."

He read all he could about GSS before his visit with Faye, outlining a clear pattern that grimly aligned with the progression he'd observed in his family members: symptoms usually arise when people are between thirty-five and fifty-five; at first they include an inability to coordinate movement, and things get steadily worse from there. Large muscles in the arms and legs contract, causing excruciating pain. Speech becomes slurred as the tongue grows more difficult to control and swallowing becomes a near impossibility. Brain deterioration can leave a patient blind or deaf. Many—though not all—become demented, but everyone meets the same end: death, usually within five years from the onset of symptoms.

The puzzle was coming together. Tim felt the cold sweat of certainty. He had to get to Faye as quickly as possible.

Tim left Clemson early in the morning when the sky was still inky dark, driving over the Smoky Mountains. He thought it would just be a short trip but he ended up driving for nearly six hours. He barely noticed the sun coming up, the muted light, the bluish mountains in the morning haze. He drove in a daze, terrified of what he'd see when he got to Huntsville. He'd brought a video camera—to this day he does not know why he thought to bring it, but he is glad he did.

It was lunchtime when Tim finally pulled up to Faye's building, parked his car, and took an elevator to her fourth-floor apartment. Faye's adopted daughter, Betsy, opened the door. Faye was behind her in a wheelchair. Tim's worst fears were confirmed when he saw her face; she had that strange, bulging-eyed stare, the exact same frozen visage he had seen with his father. Her voice was weak, she could not walk, her arms and legs were shaky. It was unmistakable. This was not Parkinson's; this was Bill's disease. This was GSS.

Tim tried to keep the realization from dawning on his face while the two said "I love you" to each other, Faye pushing the words out with difficulty. He could not keep the thought out of his mind: this disease will kill the Baxley family.

While they ate lunch, Tim gently questioned Faye. "What were your symptoms?" he asked, feeling a dagger of anxiety when she replied that the first sign had been random dizziness—she was walking down the street and suddenly felt the sidewalk spin.

When lunch was over, Tim examined Faye while Betsy's husband held the video camera, recording the process. Tim explained that the video might be important later for her diagnosis and treatment, and Faye did not object. Her chin-length brown hair with gray showing at the roots was carefully styled, swept back from her forehead in a poufy wave. But her face was expressionless, rigid. She stared straight ahead, not even glancing at Tim, who bent over her, gently examining the muscle tone in her arms and legs, giving her soft caresses, asking her if he was hurting her. His voice was comforting, and he touched her often, a hand on her shoulder, a gentle stroking of her thigh.

"I've already checked her reflexes," Tim said, looking into the camera, "and they were, uh, they were not brisk." He pointed out a strange pattern of movement, recording it on the video. "You've got kind of a circular movement you do with your hands—not intentionally," he hastened to add, as Faye, still expressionless, rubbed one thumb against the other. Don't let your alarm show, Tim told himself, don't let her see the turmoil you are feeling. But she must have been sensing it. She knew what had happened to her brother Bill. She'd talked to Mike, answered his questions when he'd called her to fill out the family tree. Faye was a rocket scientist, literally; she must understand what was happening to her.

Still, Tim knew the only way to handle the situation was with utter frankness. He had to tell Faye what he suspected, and he had to ask her if, when she died, she would agree to a brain autopsy to determine if she had the disease. After all, Tim told himself, he might not ever see Faye again. What if she died before he could ask about getting her brain? She was the family's only hope of confirming the illness.

So he explained to her what he suspected and what would happen if she agreed to an autopsy. A pathologist would cut open her skull and remove the brain and the dura, the tough bisque-colored shell covering the brain. The pituitary gland and the brain stem would be removed too, and after the pathologist had done his work, her brain would be sent off for analysis.

Faye listened carefully, then silently nodded her assent.

Tim left that afternoon, haunted on the long drive back by what he had seen, panicked about what might happen to him and his brothers.

He got home late that night and told Janet what he had

observed. She tried to reassure him. "No matter what it is," she said, "we will deal with it and get through it."

Tim went online to search for GSS experts and found a doctor, a neuropathologist named Pierluigi Gambetti, at Case Western Reserve University in Ohio. He called Gambetti, telling him he was a member of a family that had a GSS gene mutation and that he wanted to send Faye's brain and spinal cord for analysis after she died. In truth, he really had no proof the disease in his family was GSS, but he wanted to be sure Gambetti would analyze Faye's nervous system tissue. Before he said anything to his brothers, he had to get his hunch confirmed. He had to wait for Faye to die.

He got the phone call in July 2002. Betsy let him know that Faye was in the hospital, near death. It had been a year since he'd visited Faye, interviewing her and recording her movements.

Tim had to move fast now, arranging for a pathologist to come to the hospital as soon as Faye died. Her brain had to be removed before an enzyme could start chewing it up, destroying any prions. It had to go to Gambetti immediately, by Federal Express.

The pathologist would have to be willing to take the necessary precautions—donning a total body exhaust suit, to seal his body entirely from head to toe and protect him from coming into contact with Faye's brain, in case whatever she had could be transmitted. After removing the brain, the pathologist would also have to make sure his instruments were fastidiously disinfected.

Gambetti helped Tim find a pathologist in Huntsville who would do the work, and after an anxious flurry of phone calls while Faye was in the hospital, the arrangements were made. Faye died on July 12, just a few days after entering the hospital. The pathologist did his work quickly and efficiently, and the brain was shipped immediately to Case Western Reserve. Now all that was left was waiting to learn what Gambetti would discover.

A couple of weeks later, Gambetti called Tim. The antibodies he had used were marked with a fluorescent dye. If Faye had GSS, those antibodies would give off a bright light when they attached to the misfolded prions.

"Your aunt's cerebellum lit up like a Christmas tree," Gambetti told Tim, oblivious to the impact of his words. Faye had GSS.

Tim had to tell his brothers.

Tim called Billy first, proud of what he had discovered but also appalled by what it meant. Those mixed feelings festered in him as he summoned all his faculties to sound casual.

"Hey, Billy, okay if I swing by?"

Billy replied that of course it was, and Tim forced himself into his car. On the way there, he gripped the steering wheel and ran over the conversation he would have with his brother, practicing the opener as a refrain so as not to botch it.

He worried that he had to frame that conversation with Billy just right. When he arrived, he found Billy where he always was on Saturday afternoons during football season, sitting on the sofa in the living room watching a game on TV. Billy was finding it hard to walk these days—but even before, when he was healthy, he'd sit for hours watching the game.

Tim waited for a commercial, then began to speak, wasting little time before blurting out why he had come. He explained about Faye, about the antibody test, about GSS. "Billy, I am almost certain this is what it is," he told his oldest brother. Billy stared at Tim calmly. Then he asked Tim in his weak voice, "What is the next step?"

Tim did not expect this, he thought Billy would be angry,

or perhaps refuse to discuss his illness. But a different side of him emerged with this news; he was more compliant, or perhaps he was finally beaten down from battling his illness.

Tim explained to Billy that there was a blood test for the GSS gene and Case Western Reserve could do the test. Tim had found a doctor, Michael Geschwind, at the University of California in San Francisco, an expert who could examine Billy if he wanted to go there.

Billy did not reply, remaining silent for some time after that; Tim decided he'd said enough.

Billy sent his blood to Case Western Reserve immediately and got a letter telling him what he already knew by then—he had a prion gene mutation for GSS.

Then he and Steve made the arduous trip to San Francisco, where Geschwind confirmed that his disease was far advanced and there was no treatment.

Tim knew that telling Buddy would be more difficult. He was still clinging to the idea that he did not have the family disease. While it was true that insomnia is not typically associated with GSS, or at least not insomnia of such a long duration, there was another prion disease—fatal familial insomnia—that did involve sleeplessness. Still, this was caused by a different mutation in the prion gene, and it was almost inconceivable that everyone else had the GSS mutation and Buddy had the one for fatal familial insomnia. Tim didn't have an answer to that particular part of the riddle, and he did not see any reason to confront Buddy's denial of the possible significance of his symptom. But he felt convinced that Buddy's insomnia was not a good sign.

Buddy was also calm when Tim told him what he'd found. Too calm. "You know, I've been checking myself for nystagmus," he said. Only a fellow doctor, a neurologist, would get the joke. You can't check yourself for nystagmus, a rhythmic involuntary movement of the eyes—up and down or in circles or side to side—that often shows up in diseases of the brain's cerebellum. That was Buddy's way of making light of the scary situation. Tim was reminded once again that Buddy just did not believe—refused to even consider the possibility—that he had GSS.

That night, when he got home, Buddy told Kathy about Tim's call. It was so shocking that Tim had found the name of the disease that killed Faye and his father, he said—and it was almost certainly what was killing Billy. A terrible, awful disease, Buddy and Kathy told each other. But Kathy agreed with Buddy. His symptoms weren't the same as his father's and they weren't the same as Billy's. He just had a terrible case of insomnia.

Coincidentally, Buddy's insomnia ended shortly after Tim's call. He had no idea what made it finally go away, but one night he managed to sleep through until morning, and the next night it happened again. Yet as the insomnia waned, something else started to happen. He began to lose coordination in his hands.

Buddy had always had a steady hand. But one day he found he had trouble tying the knot after he stitched a patient. He did not say anything to Jane, his nurse, and she reasoned that maybe his eyesight was getting bad. Soon after, his handwriting, never good, became illegible. When he tried to pick up a pen to write a prescription his fingers would not work; he could not hold the pen. Jane began writing prescriptions for him. Buddy did not tell Kathy.

Buddy could no longer laugh off the possibility that he had GSS. He'd seen these symptoms before—in his father, in his brother—and with growing dread and certainty, he felt that his future would be no different. But maybe he was wrong, he told himself. He'd had so much stress for so many years. So much worrying over his father, then his mother who had to bear up under the terrible burden of chasing this mystery disease while her husband succumbed; so much pain, watching his brother go through it all again. Enough accumulated stress can cause even the most reliable, well-maintained machine to break down. And his problems had started differently, he reminded himself; they had started with insomnia.

Buddy began talking more slowly and with increasing effort. He began to stumble and weave as if he were drunk. He declared that he had developed supranuclear palsy, a rare and serious brain disorder that causes victims to weave and lurch. It was another agonizing disease without a treatment or cure—but it was *not* inherited. That was important to him—if he had supranuclear palsy, he could not have passed it on to his children. He and Kathy began giving money to the Supranuclear Palsy Foundation, as did their friends.

Tim saw what was happening to his brother Buddy on his visits to Hartsville. He had heard rumors that the staff at the hospital were whispering that Dr. Buddy was a drunk. He cringed when he saw the way Buddy was walking and his shaky hands. He knew the supranuclear palsy idea made little sense, but what would be the point of confronting Buddy? Let him keep his illusions a while longer, Tim thought.

On the Saturday before Christmas in 2002, five months after Faye died, Buddy and Kathy were together at home when the phone rang. It was one of Buddy's patients. Her little boy had cut himself—a three-quarter-inch gash on his upper lip—and she could not stop the bleeding. Bring him to the office, Buddy told her instinctively. But he knew he was in trouble. He could not hold a pen—how could he hold a needle if the child needed stitches?

He turned to Kathy. "You will have to help me."

Kathy and Buddy put on their coats and got into the Bronco. Kathy was shaken. He'd never asked her to come along. What was going on? They sat quietly on the short drive to the office.

When they arrived, Buddy took the little boy into an exam room. He asked Kathy to come with him to an adjacent room and confessed to her that he no longer had the strength in his hand to push a needle through a child's skin. As she sat there, stunned, he explained the procedure. "Here is what you have to do." He would tell her where to place the needle for each stitch and she would push it through. Then he would point to where the next stitch should go and she would push the needle through the boy's skin again. The main thing she had to concentrate on was making sure the line of stitches was perfectly straight.

It was hard for Kathy to take this in. She knew Buddy had struggled mightily with insomnia and now had a bit of a palsy, a little trouble walking. But she had ascribed these difficulties to the possibility of supranuclear palsy. Buddy had been putting in stitches for decades; it was something so routine he should be able to do it without thinking. Suddenly she knew that Buddy had been hiding the true extent of his disease from her. She felt bewildered and crushed. And heartbroken for her proud husband.

And she was nervous; she was not capable of putting stitches in that little boy's lip. "I don't know how hard to push," she told Buddy. "I don't know if it will hurt him."

"Push hard," Buddy replied. "It will not hurt him."

Kathy did not want to do it; she had to fight her impulse to refuse, to tell Buddy to send the child to an emergency room. But she could not do that, she could not humiliate him that way, she could not defy a man who had humbled himself before her. She knew she had to make those stitches.

Buddy and Kathy went back into the exam room where he told the boy's mother that he was a little shaky so Kathy was going to help. Buddy was composed, hiding his emotions with his gentle words. At all costs, that mother and her little boy could not know what was really going on.

Kathy was frightened as Buddy filled a syringe with Xylocaine to numb the boy's lip. Following his instructions, Kathy guided the needle for Buddy while he pushed it in, injected the drug, then pulled it out.

When the anesthetic had taken effect, Buddy told Kathy to start stitching. The fishhook-shaped needle was held by a hemostat, a tweezer-like pair of scissors that locked together. He handed the hemostat to Kathy. "I need you to do this," he said, locking eyes with her.

Kathy began, unnerved by the situation, worried that there would be a scar and that the stitches would not line up correctly. Buddy stood beside her, emanating calm. "It will be fine," he said, as she gazed up at him.

As Kathy pushed the needle into the boy's skin—so firm, so tough to puncture—Buddy spoke to the boy, soothing him, never letting on that anything was amiss. The first stitch was in. Kathy looked up at Buddy. "Okay, that's good, that's good," Buddy coached her. She pulled it through and put it in position for the next step. "That's good," he told her again, talking her through every step of the procedure.

It turned out to be much easier than Kathy had expected. But she was devastated. It was so hard, so embarrassing for her husband to step back like that. On the way home she did not say much and neither did Buddy, just small talk. But when they entered the house Kathy turned to him. "I didn't know you had this problem."

Buddy sat down; he hesitated, looking closely at Kathy before he began. Then he told her about the nurses writing prescriptions for him and the weakness in his hands, the shakiness, and how he had been trying to conceal the difficulty he experienced even when walking.

She was flooded with sorrow. She knew him so well, knew how hard it was for her husband to admit any weakness. She knew he had kept all this from her, in part because he wanted to keep his problems to himself—but another part of it was denial. Her grief was accompanied by piercing fear. It all fit together and it had nothing to do with stress, nothing to do with the troubles with Amanda. Supranuclear palsy now seemed like such an obvious ruse. In her heart, she knew this was the start of something terrible, but still she prayed there could be a different ending.

# 9

# No Return

The envelope with the Case Western Reserve return address was on the kitchen counter mixed in with advertising fliers and credit card offers. No one had bothered to look at the mail yet. Buddy, just back from the office, walked into the kitchen on that chilly day in February of 2004, inhaling the familiar odors of the dinner Kathy was cooking—meatloaf and mashed potatoes. When he saw the stack of mail, he began rifling through it. Then he saw the letter. He felt a sick sense of foreboding. Here it was: the dividing line. The before and after of Buddy Baxley's life.

He had decided to have the GSS gene test not long after that awful night when Kathy had to sew the stitches. But even as he sent in vials of his blood, he still hoped he would be spared. Sure, he was having some balance issues and his hands were weak. But he wasn't incapacitated. He thought of Billy, who was much worse off than he—maybe he didn't even have the same disease.

It had taken two months for the results to arrive, so long that Kathy had stopped examining the mail every day, waiting for the letter. Now it was here, too soon. He was not ready to open the letter, he wished for more time, more time to live in ignorance.

Buddy stood at the kitchen counter, holding the envelope,

willing himself to slit it open. He took a deep breath, exhaled, and pulled out the letter. It was just one page, a form letter—the same letter Billy had gotten a year earlier. It was not written in patient-friendly language; it was meant to go to the patient's doctor, but Buddy *was* a doctor. So the letter had come to him.

His eyes scanned the page. He looked up at his wife, and made a noise, *hmpff*, like someone had punched him in the gut. His face ashen, he grunted, "Gosh dang it."

Seeing the result written on Case Western Reserve letterhead, with its technical boilerplate language, with its advice that patients be told the result in the presence of a genetic counselor, made the unthinkable real for the first time.

Amanda, a nineteen-year-old freshman in college, happened to be home for a visit that weekend. She was sitting in the family room just off the kitchen and looked up as Buddy read the letter out loud.

She covered her mouth in shock, then started to cry. She felt broken, bereft, frightened about what was to come. Her dad did not have long to live, he had the disease that had killed her grandfather and was now killing her uncle Billy.

Buddy tried to reassure his stunned wife and daughter. "Ain't nothing but a thing," he said, meaning it was just a piece of paper. They were not going to get upset about it. They would trust in God and go on with their lives.

At some point in that evening, Amanda walked outside and looked up at the inky sky, staring at God, or whoever was watching over her and her family. "Why?" she cried. "Why *my* dad?"

And of course, as a premed major, as the daughter and niece of doctors, she realized full well what the result meant for her. She too might have the gene. She might get the family disease. She forced herself to push that thought out of her mind and concentrate on the unfolding tragedy in front of her.

The family tried to take its cues from Buddy. They would

be strong. They would continue as they had been. It would be an ordinary weekend. They told Amanda's brother, Luke, who rushed home from college. Luke had always been the golden child: popular, athletic, close to everyone in the family. He wanted to be a doctor just like his dad. Now he felt for the first time the wallop of tragedy. He and Buddy embraced and Luke wept, his voice thick as he told Buddy, "We don't have enough time."

The eldest of Buddy's children, Holly, was devastated when she heard what had happened. She turned to her strong religious beliefs for comfort. From the start, Holly had been a light in both her parents' lives. She was tall and beautiful and could always be counted on to stay out of trouble. She was an exemplary student too, so serious about her studies that she graduated from high school a year early.

In her early twenties, already married for three years to a man she had met in college, Holly had developed what she describes as "a closer relationship with Christ." Religious as her upbringing had been, she chided her parents, whom most people would have described as quite religious, for not having properly developed her relationship with Jesus. From that point forward, the Bible became her reference point and her moral compass. When Buddy got that letter, she and her husband already had one child, a baby boy. His life, she trusted, was in God's hands. She was not going to worry about whether she or her baby had inherited her father's illness.

Over the next few days and weeks, the impact of that letter hit Kathy. Everything she and Buddy had dreamed of and planned for the rest of their lives was forever altered. Buddy was her companion and her protector. She had never worried about finances—Buddy was the breadwinner. How could the family cope with what was to come. How could they even afford it?

Kathy tossed in bed at night, tormented by unanswerable questions: Do we have to sell the house? Do I keep working? Does he keep working? Their suffering is a test of sorts, Kathy decided, telling herself, "This is when you find out if your faith is real."

She and Buddy turned to God, praying together, taking comfort in a verse from Philippians. "Be anxious for nothing, but in everything by prayer and supplication, with thanksgiving, let your requests be made known to God. And the peace of God, which surpasses all understanding, will guard your hearts and minds through Christ Jesus."

Buddy, vowing to go on as usual, continued seeing patients, refusing to let the diagnosis defeat him. He could not even imagine giving up his medical practice. Being a doctor was his calling, his passion, his identity. So he continued to go to the office every day, seeing patients even as his hands shook and he lurched and swayed when he walked. Finally, after nearly two years, he admitted it to himself that it was no longer safe for him to treat patients. Even talking had become difficult. He had to retire.

His patients were distraught. If you can't stand we will hold you up, they told him. Buddy's nurse, Jane Putnam, who had seen his disease progress from a deteriorating handwriting to this, was desolate. "There's not another Buddy," she cried.

In October 2004, Buddy shuttered the office doors. Retirement was a hard adjustment. He'd once confessed to his daughter Amanda that he feared ever being a burden, telling her, "If I ever get sick, put me in a boat and push me out into the Gulf of Mexico."

He had planned to work until he was sixty-five at least, then retire and live in the dream house he and Kathy had built on a piece of property they'd been eying for years. It was beside the lake in a peaceful neighborhood near his mother's house.

Buddy had had a vision of the idyllic life he'd have there, imagining that when he quit working he'd sit on a porch swing and look out at the still water he loved so much, do a little fishing, some boating, do some skeet shooting, hunt doves and ducks, do some yard work. He'd play golf—he'd been named the most valuable player on the Hartsville High School team in 1969 but had no time for the game when he was practicing medicine. The house was taupe, two stories, with a wraparound porch, a lushly planted garden. He and Kathy had lined the driveway with dogwood trees, a Christian symbol: it is said that a dogwood was used to make the cross for the Crucifixion. They put a wreath on the door, a Jesus statue in the side yard, and, in front, a small statue of Mary on one side and St. Francis on the other.

With the news of Buddy's diagnosis, those plans were swept away. Yet Buddy tried to disguise his symptoms from his family. He did not want their pity, did not want their help. He insisted on doing yard work, even as movement became problematic.

"That is his way of still trying to live," Amanda concluded. But she was frightened by what was happening to him. Once, when Buddy was outside with a wheelbarrow, all alone, he fell into a drainage ditch in front of the house. He was there more than an hour, waving his arms, until Kathy came looking for him. Buddy laughed it off, refusing to give up working on his yard. It was a stark reminder of how bad things were and how hard Buddy had to work to conceal what was happening to him.

His balance grew worse and worse. One day he fell so precipitously in his kitchen that his head put a dent in the black metal handle of the oven door.

Now Merle had to watch her two oldest sons suffer the same fate as her husband. The only consolation, if you could call it that, was that they had grown close in their suffering. Before

GSS robbed them of their voices, they spoke on the phone regularly, bonded by their mutual journey down this strange road. When they lost the ability to talk they would come to Merle's house for a visit, sitting side by side in their wheelchairs, turning their heads toward each other and locking eyes.

Once, during one of these visits, both men suffering terribly, hardly able to walk or talk, Billy lurched up, ready to go home. Buddy lurched over to him and the two brothers embraced. Merle watched and felt her heart break.

Kathy was consumed with guilt, dreading the thought of having to take care of Buddy through the years of decline she knew were coming. She worried about what her life would become, taking care of a man who could not walk, could not talk, could not swallow? But then: How could she harbor thoughts like that about her own husband? And why was God inflicting this suffering on them?

A book called *A Grace Disguised: How the Soul Grows Through Loss* helped her with its talk of love and how to be faithful. And she clung to her Bible studies. She wrote passages from scripture and kept them in her car, flipping through them when she stopped at traffic lights.

Kathy had come to her religious convictions as a teenager. Her parents were Episcopalian, but when she was fourteen, her friend invited her to a Valentine's Day banquet sponsored by the youth group at an evangelical church. There, three young men sang of their faith and their love for Jesus.

Afterward, Kathy and her friend went to the church sanctuary where they met the young men, who told them that human beings were sinful without Christ. They told them to open their hearts to him and he would come in and clean them so that they were as white as snow, that they would be holy and filled with his holy spirit.

That night, Kathy felt something change inside of her. She

was filled with the holy spirit; she felt as white as snow. And she wanted more and more of it.

She joined a Bible study group led by a boy at her school who was one grade ahead of her. For the next four years, those weekly sessions, reading and discussing scripture, were the center of her life. She left the staid Episcopal church and joined a Baptist church with enthusiastic and vocal believers.

Her parents were concerned. Where did this religious zealotry come from? "Kathy, you are getting a bit charismatic," her mother told her.

But it was this bedrock of faith that allowed Kathy to face her situation with Buddy. She worked hard at accepting the new reality. She told herself she couldn't live a life of despair. God would show her what path to take. And, ultimately, Kathy came to feel a sense of peace and acceptance.

She was even able to untangle her fears about their financial future. Buddy had sold his practice when he retired—that was a source of money. And ten months before Buddy got sick he had, for no particular reason, doubled his life insurance. He also had disability income.

Meanwhile, Kathy kept working, managing a free medical clinic in Darlington that was supported by a group of churches and businesses. It helped so much to be able to get out of the house, to assist other people, to get away from her husband's agony.

The next year Kathy took Buddy to San Francisco to see Michael Geschwind, the doctor specializing in GSS that Tim had found. Geschwind was studying people with GSS and their family members, documenting symptoms and the ages when the disease began, looking for patterns. Billy had already joined the study. Now Buddy wanted to be part of it, to do anything he could to help doctors understand this horrible disease.

Kathy and Buddy set off in late February 2005, on a bleak

day with a biting wind. She knew it was not going to be easy for Buddy to get to San Francisco—he was still able to walk, but slowly and with a great deal of shaking and lurching. And although he could talk, it was with agonizing difficulty and his speech was hard to understand. Yet Kathy hoped, by participating in Geschwind's study, Buddy would feel lifted by making a contribution to science in this way.

Kathy helped Buddy down the wooden steps from their front porch and onto the crunchy gravel driveway where their car was waiting. She loaded in Buddy's walker and their luggage, clicked on their seat belts and drove to the airport in Florence, about forty-five minutes from their home. They climbed into a small propeller jet that would take them to the larger airport in Charlotte. Everyone was patient as Kathy helped Buddy maneuver onto the plane and into his bulkhead seat.

In the Charlotte airport, Kathy pushed Buddy in a wheelchair, pulling her luggage behind her. She bought herself her favorite Starbucks drink, a hazelnut latte. Then she headed for a restroom, parking Buddy at the door and handing him her Starbucks cup to hold. When she came out, she discovered someone had dropped money into the cup, assuming Buddy was mentally disabled and was begging. Telling Kathy what had happened, Buddy made the peculiar sound that served as laughter in those days when he had lost the use of the muscles of his tongue. It was a loud "heh" sound made as he sharply drew in breath through his mouth. Kathy laughed with him. That was Buddy, she thought. Determined to keep his pride. Better to laugh than cry.

When they arrived in San Francisco, they checked in to a hotel, a hilly mile and a half from the university's medical campus on Parnassus Avenue, a complex of tall gray buildings high above Golden Gate Park. The next morning they left for Buddy's appointment with Geschwind, slowly making the trip by foot—Buddy using his walker. A mile and a half never seemed so long. After that they took cabs, an ordeal because it took so long to get Buddy into a cab, but much better than walking.

Geschwind, a short, solid man with a rosy complexion and a kind but somewhat awkward manner, put Buddy through a series of tests—lab tests, neurological tests, and psychological tests of his memory and reasoning. At one point, he turned to Buddy and asked, "Why are you here?" Without hesitation, Buddy replied in his weak and halting voice, "To help my kids."

GSS was relentless. It was becoming increasingly clear that it was going to render Buddy a shell of the man he had been. He could feel it coming, he knew the symptoms all too well, and yet he struggled mightily against it.

The illness was ceaselessly physically demanding—there was no getting used to it, it simply happened. But there was a psychological lag time; trying to face the new reality that this illness had ushered in was like trying to imagine the true size of the universe. Buddy felt a certain amount of pride—he did not want to be remembered as a feeble, sick man, utterly dependent on others. But there was also not a small amount of denial mixed into his attitude as well—the more he could hold on to who he was, he believed on some level, the less the disease could take over his existence. He did not want to give in to GSS.

Yet as time went by, little by little, it was hard not to see that GSS was winning the battle.

In July 2005, a few months after the trip to San Francisco, Buddy's speech became almost impossible to understand, forcing him to use an alphabet board to spell out his words in order to communicate.

Around the same time, Buddy and his family went to their favorite seafood place. But Buddy gagged so badly with every

bite that he finally gave up, defeated. The family left the restaurant; there was no point in continuing the meal if Buddy
couldn't eat. When they got to their car, Buddy began to weep.
Luke turned to his father and said, "We don't care that we
don't go out to eat. We care that we get to be with you when
we eat." That was the last time the family went out to a restaurant together.

The following month, Buddy was forced to surrender to the
next phase of the disease. Kathy had made steak for dinner and
chopped Buddy's portion into minuscule pieces. Despite her
effort, Buddy choked on the tiny pieces of meat, strangling and
coughing. Kathy was terrified.

"Sweetheart," she said, "you know as a medical person that
if you inhale a piece of food it will give you pneumonia."

He nodded.

"Why don't I try processing this steak and see what it tastes
like?"

Buddy looked at her, his eyes welling, and nodded again.
He looked down at his alphabet board and spelled out "please."

From that day on, Buddy ate nothing that was not pureed.

His brother Billy, on the other hand, refused to give in on
this front. Proud and defiant, he continued to cough and choke
on his food until the day he died of pneumonia, most likely
from inhaling food.

Even with pureed food, Buddy's weight kept dropping.
Kathy stayed home from her job, hoping if she was there all
day she could fatten Buddy up. Instead, he lost fifteen pounds
in three weeks, his weight falling to 106 pounds. She decided
staying home was not helping and went back to work—leaving
him to be cared for by home health aides.

"Come on, laugh, have some fun, I said one night before
going to sleep," Kathy wrote in a journal she kept at the time.
"He mumbled something and I asked him what he said. He said,

'Can't have fun.' I asked him why and he said he can't have fun anymore. I told him I understood that it was hard. No, I didn't understand. No one could. I asked him if he was tired of everything. He said he was tired of being a burden to everyone."

Kathy wrote about her struggle to accept Buddy's illness as part of God's plan. "No, Lord, it hasn't been easy. But I'll stop asking for it to be. You said ask and you will receive. I'd like him back walking and talking but if that's not in your plan, I'm not going to stop loving you now. You've been with me all my life and you have worked some amazing miracles in my life. I won't stop believing in you now because I am so grateful. But I don't know the best you can do in this situation. I just ask that you do it. And I'll be so grateful."

As Buddy got more and more debilitated, the family vowed to make the most of his remaining time, spending days and evenings and weekends with him. The hardest thing for Holly, Luke, and Amanda was that they could no longer talk to their father on the phone. He was unable to speak.

Amanda came home from college every other weekend to help. Luke called frequently and came home from medical school as often as he could. Holly visited on the weekends when she could get away. She lived about forty-five minutes away, working as a math teacher and taking care of her little boy. During Buddy's illness she became pregnant again with another boy, trusting in God to take care of her and her family even if she had the GSS mutation.

Buddy's brother Mike, who lived in town, came nearly every day after work and read to him from Louis L'Amour novels and the collections of Archibald Rutledge, the poet laureate of South Carolina, who wrote about adventures in the woods and nature. Rutledge was one of Buddy's favorite authors—Mike read through all of his books twice.

Townspeople and former patients offered to help. Kathy's

Sunday school class at Lakeview Baptist Church began delivering meals to their house every Tuesday night, when Kathy was working nights at the medical clinic. Whenever Kathy tried to thank them, they replied it was a blessing to help.

Kathy subscribed to the western channel on cable television so Buddy could watch his favorite movies. He would spend his days in a brown leather recliner in the paneled living room, watching Clint Eastwood and John Wayne.

Life at home was hard—and getting ever harder—especially when communicating was so difficult. Buddy would get frustrated, angry with himself, waving his hands about, grunting. But he had vowed not to wallow in self-pity.

The first time Amanda helped her father use the bathroom she was nervous and embarrassed for him. Buddy was a very modest man. She wheeled him into the bathroom and picked him up. His head was resting on her shoulder—his muscles were contracted and he couldn't sit up. She put him on the commode and bent down, face-to-face, and said, "Is this okay?" He looked up. He never, ever in his life would have allowed his daughter to help him when he had a bowel movement. But when he could still talk he used to say, "You've got to laugh about it or it will drive you crazy. We are not going to cry. We are not going to get mad." That day, Buddy met his daughter's eyes and burst out laughing with his odd "heh" sound.

In 2006, Buddy's office reopened as a free medical clinic. Kathy managed it along with the clinic in Darlington. One of Buddy's patients painted his portrait and Kathy hung it on a wall in the waiting room. The family took Buddy there in a wheelchair for the opening ceremony. Buddy, with his shaking hands, managed to cut the ribbon.

Buddy died, at 1:00 a.m. on April 16, 2010. It was almost two years to the day after his brother Billy died.

Buddy, like Billy, died at home. Kathy and a hospice nurse cared for him until the end. Earlier that day, Kathy had asked the preacher at her church, "When is enough enough?"

When she heard the nurse's footsteps coming up the stairs to her room in the middle of that night, she sat up immediately.

"He's gone, isn't he?" Kathy asked. And she felt a burden had been lifted.

But an unspoken question hung over the Baxleys: Who would be next?

# 10

# Tested

Tim glanced at the chart on the wall outside the exam room in his neurology office, knocked, and walked in. The first patient of the day, an elderly man, was sitting on the narrow examination table, his wife at his side. Tim greeted the man with a friendly smile. As soon as he saw him, he knew what was wrong. Parkinson's disease. The man was shaking, trembling. Tim forcibly focused on this new patient and the diagnosis he was going to have to give him. Every time was excruciating—but even more so now that Tim himself had such a delicate understanding of the hope a person clings to when facing this kind of health crisis.

The man was surely wishing for an innocent explanation, a benign tremor, a condition that could be easily treated and cured. But all Tim could offer would be treatments to quell the symptoms temporarily as the disease took its inexorable course.

"That's my future," Tim thought. "Not decades away but a few years down the line."

His days now were filled with patients who struck him with dread. The stroke patient who had trouble talking. The woman with dizzy spells. And most of these people were elderly. Tim was only forty-two. Everything seemed to remind him. Was he a bit woozy when he stood up? Was that stumble really an accident?

He confided in his brother. "Hey, Mike," he said, "When I go around a corner quickly sometimes it seems like my right leg is slipping out. Did Billy and Buddy ever say anything to you about that?"

No, Mike replied. Billy and Buddy had not mentioned a symptom like that. "You know, Tim, that same thing happens to me sometimes," Mike answered reassuringly.

Mike, age forty-six, unmarried, had recently left his small law practice to become a judge. He too had suffered the anxiety that Tim was going through. But, unlike Tim, he couldn't stand to live in the gray area of not knowing, his nerves frayed by the uneasy questions: Did my leg just slip out from underneath me? Am I slurring my words? Is that a tremor in my hand?

Mike had gotten a blood test a couple of years earlier, in 2002, soon after Tim told him there was one available at the National Prion Disease Pathology Surveillance Center at Case Western Reserve University.

He knew he had to plan his life. Who would want to be in a courtroom presided over by someone who appeared drunk, with an unsteady gait and slurred speech? Who would want a judge with handwriting so shaky it was illegible? And how could he work if GSS also robbed him of his ability to think and remember?

So he was the first to be tested. Two months went by, an unbearable time to wait. Every time his phone rang, Mike leapt to answer it, wondering if it would be his doctor calling with the result.

Finally, he got a voicemail from his doctor's office asking him to make an appointment and come in. Mike went cold with dread. If the news was good, wouldn't his doctor have just picked up the phone and called him? His heart pounding, he called back. His doctor came on the line right away. The test was negative, he said. Mike did not have GSS.

Mike sat at his desk, alone in his office, exhaled, and then began to weep, his relief tinged with a sense of injustice. The thought went through his mind: Buddy saved peoples' lives. He put them in prison. Why should Buddy be the one to die?

Tim was reassured when he spoke to Mike that day, at least about his leg slipping. If it happened to Mike, and Mike did not have the mutated gene, then that symptom, at least, was not the start of GSS. Tim knew he could end the suspense at any time, as Mike had done, by sending his blood in to be tested for the mutation. But he just could not bring himself to do it. His plan had been to live his life as though he was not going to get GSS, but that was proving to be harder than he had ever imagined.

Two terrible years went by with him half-believing the symptoms of GSS had begun—but too paralyzed by indecision to find out the answer for real. He confided in his pastor and close friend, Von Reynolds, a small man with soft white hair, wire-rimmed glasses, a dimpled smile, and a gentle manner. Von looked at Tim and listened carefully but did not tell Tim what to do.

One crisp fall evening in 2004, a year after his brother Buddy had gotten that envelope from Case Western Reserve confirming his diagnosis, Tim and Von and their two families met at a popular barbecue restaurant just outside of town. Everyone got in line for the buffet, Tim and Von at the front. The two men took their loaded trays to a secluded corner table for a private conversation, sitting across from each other in a dimly lit booth. Von spoke in a hushed voice.

He and his wife Gloria were worried before their daughter Liz was born. They had just had a son with Down syndrome and Gloria was over age thirty-five when she got pregnant with Liz, increasing her risk for having another baby with the condition. They would never have had an abortion—their Southern Baptist religion forbid it—and they loved their affected son. But still, they wanted to know—they felt they needed to know. They prayed over the question and decided to get a prenatal diagnosis with amniocentesis, "to be prepared," Von told Tim.

Before Tim could say anything, Gloria and Liz, now sixteen years old, and Tim's wife and daughters came over to them, bearing their trays of food, and sat down. The moment was past. But Von's words kept circling in Tim's mind. "To be prepared." That was what he wanted, wasn't it? To be prepared in case he had the GSS gene? Didn't he want to be sure his affairs were in order for his family? To be sure he had long-term care insurance and enough life insurance to take care of his family? Didn't he want to prepare Janet for a husband who would need constant attention, who would choke on food, who could not lift himself out of his wheelchair and onto his bed at night?

And what about his daughters? They were still so young, just five and four. He thought of them in their beds at night, sweet-smelling from their baths, waiting for him to read them a book. He thought of them trudging off to school each morning, little backpacks slung over their shoulders. When do you tell children that their father will start stumbling and falling, that soon he will not be able to read to them or hold them?

He needed to be prepared. He needed to be tested.

Soon afterward, Tim and his family went to Hartsville

for a visit. Buddy and Billy came too, with their families, and so did Mike, everyone gathering at Merle's house, as in the old days. But their father was dead and Buddy and Billy were so ill.

Tim's eyes kept drifting toward his mother. "Her two first-born sons," he thought to himself. "She raised them, changed them, watched them grow and play together. And now she is watching them die together."

He spoke to his brother Buddy about how he was holding up. Buddy, Tim learned, was taking comfort from a book called *The Giving Tree.* "That tree gave everything," Buddy said. He saw the story—in which an apple tree gave all it had to a little boy, continuing to give as the boy grew up until finally, when the boy returned as an old man, nothing was left of the tree but a stump, which provided a place for the boy to rest—as a parable about the joy of giving and about the way God would take care of him. The book, Buddy told Tim, was about unconditional love. Tim bought *The Giving Tree* later that day.

Sunday evening, back at home in Clemson, Tim gathered his two little girls—Beth, born months after his father's death, and Lee—around him and started to read them the book. Then he started to cry. Everything hit him at once. Billy and Buddy's illness, Merle's putting on a brave face, an entire family at risk.

Beth and Lee hugged their father and patted his back, not knowing what was wrong.

In the early spring of 2005, a few months after that dinner conversation with Von Reynolds, Tim steeled himself to do it, to have the blood test. He had to know if he had the GSS gene.

One evening at the hospital, Tim pulled aside his friend,

Paul Thompson, a gastroenterologist who lived next door to Tim and his family. "I need to speak to you in private," Tim said. The men went into an empty patient room, where Tim told Paul that he wanted a blood test for GSS. Tim had told him about the disease in his family and had introduced him to Billy and Buddy. Paul understood the magnitude of this task.

Then Tim waited, and waited. Once he decided to be tested, he wanted the results immediately. The way he would learn his results—with a near–form letter in the mail, just as Buddy and Billy and Mike had—was bleak, but then there was no protocol for offering people news like this, information that would so starkly change their lives.

Finally, on a spring day in 2005, Paul came by Tim's house and handed him the letter from Case Western Reserve. Then he quietly turned around and walked home.

Tim carried the letter into the back bedroom, sat on his bed, gingerly slid the letter out of its sealed envelope, and began to read. The letter was addressed to Paul:

> Dear Dr. Thompson, Jr.,
> Thank you for sending the blood sample of your patient George Timothy Baxley.
> The patient has **no mutations** in the prion protein gene. . . . Since the results of these analyses are quite complex, we strongly encourage that they be interpreted, and communicated to the family, by a genetic counselor and/or other health care professional with experience in genetic disease.
> Thank you again for sending us this interesting case.

Tim's wife Janet waited a minute before easing into the bedroom. She found her husband on his knees, weeping and praying. She felt herself go weak, sure that this meant the test was positive. "Why me?" he asked her through his tears.

His two little girls crept in, worried by the sound of their father crying. They put their arms around him and patted his back, too young to know that they had been spared.

*Part II*

# Amanda Baxley:
# The Next Generation

# 11

# A Life Transformed

On that late afternoon in February 2004, on that awful day that Buddy learned that he did indeed have GSS, Amanda looked at the waning sun glinting off the lake behind her parents' house and was hit with the stark reality of her father's disease. Her illusions, her irrational hopes that her father would somehow get better, had been stripped away in an instant when Buddy read aloud from the letter with his test results.

How unfair, she thought. She and Buddy had clashed for so long during her rebellious high school years. She hadn't even liked him very much. But in this past year things had changed. She had grown up, gotten serious about school. And she and her father had developed a special bond.

Buddy called Amanda at least once a week just to hear her voice. "Moon, how are you?" he would say when she picked up the phone, using her childhood nickname. They'd talk about her classes and he'd always ask if she had met a special guy yet. She was studying biology and planned to be a doctor. That made him so proud.

Now, just as she and Buddy had finally gotten close, Amanda and her father were going to be ripped apart by this disease.

And although it seemed almost selfish to think of it at a time like this, Amanda worried about her own future. As a premed biology major she knew how inheritance worked—each gene is present in two copies. A child inherits one copy of each gene from each parent. Buddy had one mutated prion gene and one normal one, but that one mutated gene was enough to cause the disease. Amanda knew there was a fifty-fifty chance that the prion gene she inherited from her father was the mutated one. That meant there was a fifty-fifty chance she would get GSS.

That day marked the start of a separate life for Amanda—another story. Before, she was a carefree college student, social chairwoman of her sorority, studying hard all week and partying every weekend. After, she began a different routine: study all week and then climb into her lime green Volkswagen Beetle—her parents' high school graduation present—and drive two and a half hours to Hartsville to see her parents for the weekend, helping Kathy care for Buddy. She would listen to Louis Armstrong's version of "What a Wonderful World"—her dad loved that song and it always reminded her of him. And she would be prepared with anecdotes to amuse him and medical questions from her courses that he could help her answer.

She soon dropped out of her sorority—she no longer fit in with the other girls, whose carefree lives suddenly seemed frivolous. Life had abruptly become a lot more serious for her.

When the weekend ended, Amanda always felt relieved to be leaving that house of sorrow. Back in her car, she'd play the Louis Armstrong song again. And she would be reminded of the shadow over her life.

She and her siblings would deal with the threat of GSS in different ways, and it would shape their relationship in years to come. Each had to decide if they wanted to be tested for the GSS mutation and what they would do if they had it. Holly was already married, with one child and another on the way. But Amanda and Luke were still single: If they had the test and it showed they had the gene, would they marry? Could they ask a spouse to take care of them for years only to watch them die in middle age? Was it fair to bring children into the world?

In the summer of 2005, Luke began medical school at the Medical University of South Carolina, where Amanda was an undergraduate. Although classes did not formally start until August, Luke had been invited to start in June. Every year a small group of entering medical students was picked to arrive early and take gross anatomy.

The course consisted of an activity that was considered a rite of passage in medical school—dissecting a human cadaver. Students did the dissection in teams; Luke was assigned to work with a slender, dark-haired young man named Brad Kalinsky. Quiet and reticent, socially awkward but with an electric grin that he shared with his fraternal twin Ryan, Brad soon became Luke's closest friend at medical school.

Every day for a month, Luke and Brad put on scrubs and stood over the body they were dissecting, laid out on a stainless steel table in a cold room. They shared a discomfort with the procedure and tried not to pay attention to the cloying smell of formaldehyde, standing back from this stiff naked corpse of an elderly man.

They found themselves meeting at the cadaver lab late at night to finish a dissection or test each other's knowledge of body parts. Alone in the frigid room, they began chatting about their lives, confiding among the dead bodies. Luke told his friend about his father Buddy, how he'd been a fixture in the town as the doctor who turned nobody away. And one night, he went further, glancing up from a dissection and remarking in a seemingly offhand way, "My dad has a bad neurologic disease that is untreatable."

"That sucks," Brad said.

They continued to work together in silence.

The official start of medical school, in August, began with the traditional white coat ceremony, when new medical students are presented with short white lab coats to symbolize their conversion from layperson to members of the medical profession. Amanda was there along with Buddy and Kathy to see Luke in the ceremony. After the reception, Luke approached Brad; he wanted him to meet his father. He was proud of his father; and, yes, Buddy was sick, but Luke did not want GSS to define him. He wanted Brad to see the father he had tried to portray in their conversations, the kind and compassionate doctor.

But Brad could only see what was before him, and that was a sick, feeble man who could barely keep himself upright. He was taken aback. He had envisioned Buddy as an archetypical family doctor, armed with a cracking black leather doctor's bag and sage anecdotes about making house calls in a sleepy southern town. Luke had not told Brad about Buddy's symptoms— all Brad knew was that Buddy had been forced to retire because of his neurological disease. He had not expected this frail man propped up in a walker, unable to stand or walk without assistance, his face immobile, almost masklike, though still with a hint of pride in his eyes.

"Nice to meet you, sir," Brad said. Feeling uncomfortable, he quickly walked away.

Later that semester, Brad and Luke were placed together in a small group again for a neuroscience class, just a couple of dozen students. Brad's brother, Ryan, was in the group too.

They got their assignment: each student was to give a presentation about a neurological disease. Luke had chosen GSS.

He spoke in the nondescript classroom and formally discussed the disease's clinical symptoms, its pathology, and its inheritance. How odd to be giving a talk about a disease affecting your own father, Brad observed, speaking in such a clinical way about an illness that must be causing such heartbreak.

Brad looked around the room at the other students. They seemed attentive but disengaged. It was as if there were two stories playing out. There was the serious medical student, giving a technical talk about a rare disease, one for the textbooks. And there was the hidden message beneath. This talk was really about Luke's father.

Then Brad saw the dark-haired girl in the back of the room: Amanda, Luke's sister. He had seen her briefly a few times at study sessions at Luke's house, but she'd kept out of the way. This time, though, Brad looked at her intently. He noticed she was diligently taking notes. "Why is she here?" he wondered. Maybe she was trying to impress the medical students.

Amanda did not see Brad looking back at her that day—she knew how thoroughly Luke had researched the disease so she had attended the class to learn as much as she could—but she did notice him a few weeks later when she walked into the house near the university that she shared with Luke and saw him as if for the first time. He was taking part in a study group in their living room. She immediately felt herself drawn to him, his dark good looks, his warm brown eyes; he was so attractive, she thought, and she loved his modest demeanor.

She didn't actually meet Brad until a few weeks after that, at a med school party at a rooftop bar in town. When she and Luke walked into the room, she spotted Brad immediately among the crowd of about a hundred people. He was standing against a wall with his brother Ryan.

After sipping a couple of glasses of white wine to bolster her courage, Amanda approached Brad and started a conversation by making what she knew was a lame twin joke. "Hey, I know there are two of you, but how do you tell yourselves apart?" Although they were fraternal twins, many people thought Brad and his brother looked almost identical. Ryan and Brad chuckled and Amanda started babbling, keeping a conversation going. Then she and Brad walked to the bar, sat on stools. Amanda hoped Brad was attracted to her, but he was hard to read. That social awkwardness. What did it mean?

Gathering her courage, she looked closely at Brad and said, "Want to have dinner some time?" She wrote down her phone number on a slip of paper and handed it to him, saying, "I am not going to call you. If you want to go out, call me."

Three weeks went by. "I guess he's not going to call me," Amanda thought. "I guess we didn't connect."

But then Brad did call and invited her to an expensive restaurant. They both were a bit uncomfortable as they sipped wine and ordered lamb shoulder that evening, feeling sophisticated on the one hand—their schedules and their meager spending money didn't often allow for this kind of meal—and awkward on the other, in that first-date way.

Another three weeks went by before Brad asked her out again. This time they had sushi—Amanda ordered eel for the first time, encouraging Brad to try it too. He pretended to like it. This time they felt more natural together, laughing and joking, smiling at each other warmly.

Soon after that Brad and Amanda became inseparable. He loved Amanda's adventurous spirit. She loved his kindness—it reminded her of her father's gentle nature. She also liked the reason he had chosen to specialize in nephrology, with patients whose kidneys were failing: "Usually as a doctor you see patients decline," he told her, "but here you take patients who would have been dead and bring them back from the brink, back to life."

\* \* \*

All along the issue of whether to get tested for GSS was weighing on Amanda and her brother Luke.

"I don't know what to do," Amanda told him. "I don't think I can live the rest of my life without knowing." The good news from their uncles Mike and Tim—both had tested negative for the disease—had bolstered Amanda's confidence. It gave her a flickering sense that maybe she was free of the illness too.

"I don't think I want to find out," Luke replied; despite his obsession with the illness, he'd questioned the wisdom of finding out a terrible fate years before it would happen. He knew Amanda was probably right—that eventually they'd have to face facts—but they were young yet. Why let GSS rob them of more time than need be? If he was going to get the test, he wanted to do it with more of his life under his belt.

One day, when Luke was visiting his parents, sitting on the back porch, looking out at the lake, his dad in a wheelchair beside him, he confessed his terror about the disease, his unwillingness to find out if he had it. He stared at the lake, not quite daring to meet Buddy's eyes. Buddy turned to him. "You don't have it," he said.

"How can you possibly know that?" Luke replied.

"I just know," Buddy assured him.

Of course, Luke knew his father could not really intuit if he had the mutated gene, but he clung to this conversation anyway, telling himself maybe he had escaped his father's fate.

Amanda returned to school the following year, in September 2006, and her routine continued—Hartsville and Buddy on the weekends, Brad and studies during the week.

She and Brad spoke openly about GSS. She had told him about Buddy's frightening descent into helplessness. Brad knew all too well that if he stayed with Amanda he might end up as her caregiver. And any children they had might inherit the gene too. But they never broached the topic. Amanda never asked Brad why what might be coming did not scare him off and he did not offer an explanation. The unstated assumption was that their deep love for each other would allow them to get through whatever happened. Meanwhile, they tried to go on with their lives, and their ever-deepening relationship, without dwelling on the overwhelming question: Did Amanda have the gene?

Amanda began to wonder if she had made the right choice in deciding to be a doctor. She thought of her dad's life and how often caring for his patients had taken him away from his family. She saw how much time Luke was spending studying, with many more years ahead of him even after he graduated from medical school. There would be residency, internship, perhaps years more of specialty training. She knew that more than anything she wanted to have children, and she wondered if it was possible to be the sort of deeply involved, engaged mother she hoped to be and pursue a career as a doctor.

She told Buddy about her dilemma. "I want to be there for my kids," she said. "I want to experience things with them. Is it possible to be a good doctor and a good mom at the same time?"

Buddy told her in his feeble voice, using the alphabet board when speech failed, that he would support whatever she decided to do. But he emphasized how much time a medical practice takes.

Amanda thought it over. She knew medicine would never be so important to her that she would push her children aside to focus on her career. And of course she was going to have children. She pondered the alternatives and decided to scale down her ambitions. She would become a nurse practitioner. It seemed a reasonable—and fulfilling—solution. She liked touching people, she wanted to connect with patients, and as a nurse she'd have more opportunities to get close to patients than she would as a doctor. There was a highly selective accelerated nursing program at her college. If she worked really hard, she might get in. Then she would take another year and study to be a nurse practitioner.

Brad was fine with her decision—but then he had something else occupying his mind: his relationship with Amanda. He worried it was getting too serious. Both sets of parents were opposed for religious reasons: Amanda was Southern Baptist Christian and Brad was Jewish. Despite his deepening commitment—and his ability to withstand the uncertainty of Amanda's future health—the pressure from his parents to break off the relationship and his own uneasiness about their religious differences had started to get to him. It was easier for Amanda. Kathy let her know she had difficulty at first accepting the idea that her daughter was in love with a Jewish man, but taking care of Buddy was soaking up all of her emotional energy and she did not want to take on this battle. "I just want you to be happy," she finally said to Amanda.

Brad's mother, though, was determined to stop their relationship. Her son was to marry a Jewish woman. Period. And she didn't hide her feelings from Amanda: "You are not what I imagined for my son," she told her. And then she made clear that she wasn't just talking about religion. Amanda knew that most mothers would not want their sons to marry someone who might get GSS. She herself would probably be no different if the tables were turned. But Brad's mother's words stung: "If my son marries you he has the possibility of being a widower at an early age. That is not what I want for my son."

Confronted with his mother's opposition, Kathy's discomfort, and his own concerns, Brad told Amanda they had to break up.

It lasted all of two days.

Their reunion was joyous for Amanda—she'd been devastated at the thought of living without Brad—but it also felt tentative. Though Brad returned to Amanda, making clear he couldn't live without her, the strain of their religious differences lingered. Despite the looming threat of GSS, it was the difference in their religions that caused Brad to hold back from a deeper commitment. For the time being, though, they focused on the relief of being back together, and Amanda wanted to move forward with her career plans.

In 2007, she enrolled in the accelerated nursing program at the Medical University of South Carolina—she would graduate after sixteen months, in December 2008. But her troubles weighed heavily on her: her father, the family disease, her own potential risk, her relationship with Brad, his hesitancy about marriage. It was almost too much to bear. She started seeing David Downie, a therapist. Her father had often sent young patients to him, and talking to him helped lighten the burden for Amanda. But there was always a dark shadow of despair and nothing could banish it completely.

Meanwhile, Brad finished medical school and began a residency at Vanderbilt University in Nashville. He and Amanda spoke on the phone often and visited each other when they could. But Amanda had told Brad with resolute determination that she would not move to Nashville unless he made a commitment to her.

One weekend, on a trip to Hartsville, Amanda heard an ad on her car radio for an organization called ONE that fights hunger and poverty in Africa. She focused on those two words, *hunger* and *poverty.*

"Yes," she thought. "This is it. This is what I want to do." If she went to Africa, where people were poor and hungry, she could use her nursing training to help people who really needed her. Even if it was just for a short time, it would get her out of the endless cycle of "What next?" As in, where was her relationship with Brad going? Would he marry her? And, more distressingly, when would she make a decision about getting tested for GSS? What was the next phase of the downward spiral for her father? When is this all going to end? She wanted something else to think about—a different extreme circumstance to take her out of this one.

As soon as Amanda returned to Charleston, she went online and found a group called African Impact that arranges for volunteers to work in medical clinics. She could go for a month; she could make a real difference in peoples' lives. Of course, she would have to pay her way, and that was an issue. With Buddy so sick, no longer working, requiring a paid nursing aide, her parents had no money to spare. And although she was getting to the end of her training to be a nurse practitioner, she still was a student, deeply in debt from paying for school tuition.

Going to Africa would cost $4,500, which would cover her airfare, meals, and lodging. But $4,500 might as well have been a million dollars. Still, she resolved to find a way. Her days were full, with classes and studying all week in order to free her weekends for those trips to see her parents. A part-time job was not an option. She hated the thought of putting out a call for donations and it seemed so iffy to rely on people's charity. She needed something she could do in spare moments that would bring in some money.

She finally hit upon a way that might work, although it would be time-consuming. She'd learned to make earrings from a woman at a crafts store in town. She enjoyed doing it and she was good at it too. The materials for a pair of earrings cost 50 cents. What if she charged $3 or $4 a pair and put them on cards and sold them to nursing school classmates? Kathy, who was by then managing two free medical clinics, said she would display earrings so the staff and clients could buy them.

So Amanda started making earrings in every spare moment—in the evenings after classes, at home with her parents on weekends, in breaks between classes. Kathy spoke about Amanda's quest to a local newspaper, which did a story about it, reporting that Amanda was going to Africa to honor her father, as it had always been a dream of his to do such a trip. Another local paper noticed and wrote its own story. People started sending in donations, as much as $50 and $100. Even Brad pitched in and made some earrings.

A year later, Amanda had the money. After she graduated from nursing school that December she planned to go to Africa for a few weeks at the start of the new year, in 2009.

But another, more significant, reason for the trip had emerged too. Amanda had finally made up her mind. She decided she could not live with the uncertainty of not knowing if she had the mutated gene. It had been gnawing at her, becoming an obsession. She was the kind of person who liked to make plans. She had to find out. She was going to be tested for GSS—and while she waited for the results she would be in Africa helping people. She felt it was the perfect way to spend that unbearable period between being tested and finding out.

Before the trip to Africa, then, she would go to San Francisco, undergo all the testing for Geschwind's study, and, while there, she would ask them to draw her blood and test it for GSS.

When she told Brad he immediately made it clear that he was opposed to the testing—he felt it was better not to know. If she was positive it would cast a pall over their relationship. How could they live with the knowledge that GSS was going to take her away? But he had not yet asked her to marry him, and that fall, in 2008, he had moved to Nashville to start his residency in nephrology at Vanderbilt. She could not let his wishes rule her life.

Her mother was opposed too. At the very least, she told Amanda, she should wait until Buddy died. They were suffering so much now. If Amanda were positive the burden would be just too great for Kathy to bear. And it would break Buddy's heart if he knew he had passed this disease on to her.

Amanda also told Buddy, who, unable to speak, looked at her and wept.

But once she'd made up her mind, Amanda could not be dissuaded. Ultimately, Brad and Kathy told her that, although they wished she had decided otherwise, they supported her. It was her decision. And since she had convinced herself that she did not have the GSS gene, getting tested, Amanda decided, would leave her free to live her life. She looked just like her mother, nothing at all like those Baxley men. That had to be a good sign. And Mike and Tim did not have the gene—that had to be a good omen too, didn't it?

# 12

# Options

About three hours into the five-hour cross-country flight to San Francisco, sitting in a narrow seat with no room to stretch her legs, Amanda was starting to feel ill. The pilot had warned there might be turbulence as the plane plowed into a winter storm, and sure enough, every so often the plane bucked violently and wobbly flight attendants shooed people to their seats. At least she had an aisle seat and Brad, placid Brad, was next to her, watching a movie.

She was looking straight ahead, trying to keep her anxieties at bay, when she noticed the middle-aged blind man a few rows ahead, with his dark glasses and white cane. He was pushing himself up from his seat and heading up the aisle, holding on to the backs of seats to keep his balance. He stumbled almost immediately when the plane lurched, and then he fell.

People stared, but no one made a move to help him. By instinct—was it her nursing training or years of helping her father?—Amanda leapt to her feet. She ran to the man and knelt beside him. "Hey, are you okay, sir?" she asked. He replied that he was fine, just trying to get to the lavatory.

"My name is Amanda," she said, "and I will help you."

She helped him get up, then lightly grasped the man's elbow and guided him up the aisle to the lavatory. "I will wait for you here," she said. When he came out, she guided him back to his seat.

The man turned his face toward her before he sat down. "Thank you for your kindness," he said, unable to see her but still conveying his gratitude.

Amanda walked back to her seat, bowed her head, and started to cry, so sad that she was the only one to help that man. Everyone, she thought, deserves dignity and respect. When the man fell, Brad had been turned away, staring at the movie screen. Now, as Amanda flopped back into her seat, he turned to her, concerned by her tears, and asked, "What just happened?"

She wept the rest of the trip, her emotions on edge. Her faced burned with fury at those other passive passengers, who stared as the blind man lay in the aisle.

Her thoughts drifted to her father and her uncle Billy before him. She could see them so clearly, on a plane just like this, making this same trip, Billy with his partner, Steve, and her father with her mother. She pictured her father telling her mother that he wanted to go to the lavatory, barely able to speak, trying to walk with his trembling limbs and lurching gait as Kathy tenderly held him up, guided him. No. It was too awful to even contemplate, but she could not shut off her churning imagination, could not force her mind out of that spiral of nightmarish thoughts. Now Billy was dead and her father seemed to be nearing the end too. Communicating with him had become close to impossible—it was not clear he even understood much that was going on. Kathy was still caring for him, with the help of aides, but everyone was thinking the same thing—that he and they had suffered enough. Death would be a blessed relief. When she got the results of her blood test, she'd learn whether this same fate awaited her.

And would Brad be there for her? She really did not know.

He was accompanying her to San Francisco, but the religion issue was still festering while they lived in separate cities—he in Nashville, she in Charleston. Brad knew Amanda wanted a commitment, but he kept delaying, struggling with his own conflicting emotions.

He told Amanda he was worried about how to bring up children. Both wanted children but what sort of religious education would their children have? What would they do at holidays?

Amanda answered naively: "If we love each other that's enough. We will figure out a way."

Then there was GSS. What if she had the gene? "I will be a widower very early unless a cure is found, and that doesn't look likely," Brad would say, to which Amanda would reply, "There is nothing I can do about that. It's your choice, your decision. I will understand if this is not the life you want."

Around and around they went, circling the same issues. And now they were reaching a point of no return. Amanda was going to be tested and they would know. She would have the gene. Or not.

When the plane finally landed, Amanda was glad for the distraction of figuring out how to get to their hotel. They had decided to take a subway instead of a taxi—Geschwind's grant only paid for airfare, nothing more. It would be an adventure, they told each other—they'd never taken a subway. They followed the signs in the airport and found the subway station, but it took them a while to puzzle over the maps and figure out how to buy their tickets and slip them into the turnstiles. They laughed at their confusion. "Hey, we're from the South," Amanda smiled, looking up at Brad. "We don't have subways."

They got confused again when they got out of the subway station and had to transfer to a bus. Finally, the bus let them off about a half mile from the hotel. But as they trudged up and down the steep hills, tugging their luggage, their joyful mood shattered. Amanda and Brad barely glanced at each other, somber with the same unspoken thought. How did Buddy ever negotiate this unforgiving terrain?

Amanda awoke the next morning feeling an intense, dizzying exhaustion. Did she even sleep? She was nervous and anxious, of course, but there was also a problem with their tiny hotel room and its thin walls. She and Brad could hear the people next door as if they were in the same room with them—and their neighbors had spent the night having noisy, uproarious sex. Amanda and Brad giggled at first as their neighbors went at it, but after a while they tired of hearing the noise. It made it impossible to sleep.

They had planned to start their trip by taking a couple of days to see San Francisco. Just being in that sunny city beside the sparkling bay and the bright blue sky, the crisp air, lifted their spirits on that first morning. They loved the city's eclectic neighborhoods, the diversity of the people they saw. They exclaimed with delight at the lush greenery and flowers in Golden Gate Park, at the pastel Victorian houses, the tawny hills in the distance. They took a bus to the bay and walked across the Golden Gate Bridge, looking down at the ferries and at Alcatraz prison. For brief moments, they were just like every other tourist taking in the magical city. But those moments passed. They looked at each other. Amanda voiced what they both were feeling: "You know, this really isn't a vacation."

Their mission loomed over them, and as much as they wanted to relish their visit to the city, it was a relief in a way when the time finally came to go to the university and start the testing. On the morning of their third day in the city, they headed out of their little hotel and walked over the steep hills to Geschwind's office at the University of California at San

Francisco. Amanda knew Geschwind from those two meetings of the CJD Foundation and had formed a bond with him, even going out for a drink with him and others one evening. But this was something new. Now she was a research subject and, depending on what the blood test showed, possibly a patient.

She had expected a quiet office, with almost no one around. After all, prion diseases were so rare. How many people could possibly be working on them? Instead, she saw tightly packed cubicles with more people than she had ever imagined staring at computers or typing on their keyboards. Papers and journals were everywhere, on desks and tables. Only Geschwind had a private office; his desk too was strewn with papers. He looked up and smiled when Amanda and Brad entered. For Geschwind, this was no ordinary patient visit. He remembered Amanda's uncle Billy, remembered her father, remembered talking to her at those CJD Foundation meetings. And he fervently hoped he would not have to give her bad news if she had the gene test. He had tried to develop the art of giving people bad news, but it was exhausting, so difficult. He had dealt so often with people who came to him wanting to hear they had been spared only to learn that they had a prion disease. Patients had sometimes lashed out at him. He had spent too many nights ruminating on what, if anything, he might have said or done differently. Amanda would not react with fury if she had the GSS mutation, he was sure of it, but how terrible if this vibrant young woman was destined to get the disease.

Geschwind was much more in his element when having a dispassionate discussion of the science of prions, and Amanda and Brad were only too happy to comply. Almost as soon as they sat down, they started asking questions. What does it mean to have a prion gene mutation? How does a prion gene mutate? What are your thoughts on how to cure the disease?

Geschwind looked down and fished a blank piece of paper

from the pile of journals scattered over his desk. He leaned toward Brad and Amanda, pushing the sheet of paper toward the edge of his desk so they could see it, and began drawing pictures, showing Amanda and Brad where the prion gene was located, where the tiny mutation was situated, drawing the chain reaction of twisted and distorted prion proteins that cause the disease. He told them what he hoped might come of his study. He wanted to find the very earliest signs of prion disease in order to try to stop the illness before it had a chance to irreversibly damage the brain. But when a treatment was found, it would be important not to administer it too early. All drugs have side effects and a prion drug would be doing something to proteins in the brain. It would be best to take it when prions were starting their brain-strangling chain reaction, when the benefits of the drug might outweigh any risks.

It was not clear what the normal function of prion proteins are, Geschwind confided to Amanda and Brad, but no one wanted to destroy a protein the brain needs. Studies in mice, though, had indicated that perhaps the brain can do without its usual supply of normal prions. So one idea for treatment was to block most of the normal prions so they could not start turning into those aberrant forms. Another idea was to somehow fish out or destroy the abnormal forms. Geschwind drew more pictures. He took his time, never seeming worried about keeping to a schedule.

When he'd answered all of their questions and explained the tests Amanda would undergo in the next few days, Geschwind introduced Amanda and Brad to a genetic counselor. The main concern for most genetic counselors then was with prenatal testing—older pregnant women were starting to have amniocenteses to look for abnormal chromosomes in their fetuses, with abortion as a legal option in the worst case. Genetic counselors were trained to bridge the gap between doctors and patients, explaining what results like trisomy 21, the abnormal chromosome that causes Down syndrome, meant and counseling couples who had to decide whether to continue a pregnancy. Counselors had to be a combination of psychologist and medical expert, explaining the issues in a nonjudgmental way so that patients could make up their own minds and follow their own moral codes.

But as scientists began finding genes that caused illnesses like Huntington's disease and GSS, the role of genetic counselors became more complicated. They now had to help people to understand the consequences of genetic tests that could reveal a disease that would not occur until adulthood. Frequently, counseling is left to doctors who, in surveys, confess they often do not feel prepared to discuss these issues with patients. By insisting on counseling, Geschwind's clinic was exemplary—Geschwind developed his elaborate protocol based on his instincts and on a procedure that had been developed for another disease, Huntington's—and Amanda and Brad appreciated it, difficult as it was to hear the options laid out so baldly.

Their counselor, Patricia See, was in her midthirties, Amanda estimated, and engaging, with a gentle manner as she asked probing questions.

"I know your basic story, but I want to hear it from you," See told Amanda. "I want to know why you are here."

Amanda looked up at See, gathering her thoughts. "There is a requirement that I see you and talk to you before I can get genetic testing," she said. "I know this test is going to be a big deal, and I need some genetic counseling. I need to know the best way to handle the results, whatever they are, and I want to talk about the options. If I am positive, I want to get referrals to an adoption agency."

She and Brad had already discussed the adoption option—even though he had not yet asked her to marry him, their conversations kept veering in that direction. And Brad had seen Buddy; he knew about Billy and Faye and Amanda's grandfather Bill. He knew what GSS could do to a person, to a family. Adoption seemed better than taking a chance with his children and GSS.

See seemed unperturbed by the emotional turmoil of the couple in front of her.

"What will you do if you are positive?" she asked Amanda. "Or if you are negative? How will it affect your life?"

Amanda did not hesitate. She fixed her eyes on the counselor. "If I am positive I will not take things for granted, I will live every day to the fullest," Amanda said. "If I am negative? That would be great, although I would feel guilty because my dad had to have it and my sister and brother could have it."

"What is one of your main concerns?" See continued.

"If I am positive, I am not having my own children," Amanda replied.

"Really? Why is that?"

"Because I am not going to risk passing it on."

"You have some options," See told her.

"Yeah, I know. There's adoption. That's what I am going to do," Amanda replied.

"You could take a chance and get pregnant and have the fetuses tested in utero," See suggested.

"Absolutely not," Amanda shot back. "I am not going to abort."

"There is also a new developing science, called IVF with PGD—preimplantation genetic diagnosis," See informed Amanda and Brad. "Have you heard of it?" Neither of them had. She explained: it would mean having Amanda's eggs fertilized in a petri dish—that is the IVF. Afterward, an embryologist would pluck a few cells from each embryo, which could be done without hurting them, and would test them for the

GSS mutation. Embryos with the mutation would be discarded; she could use the rest to get pregnant. The method had been used for other genetic disorders, but not yet for a prion disease. It was thought to be extremely reliable if done by experienced people.

Brad chimed in before Amanda could say anything. "Hmm," he said. "That's a lot to consider. But PGD could be a way around Amanda's abortion reservations."

Amanda remained silent, but she was not convinced: PGD sounded like abortion to her. Looking first at Brad and then at Patricia See, she spoke her mind. "It would be killing the ones that have it," she said.

She'd been brought up in a religion that believes life begins at conception and that it is unacceptable to destroy human life. There was no getting around it if you start with that premise. PGD created a real moral dilemma: for Amanda, an embryo, even one that is just a few days old, is human life.

See handed Amanda the name and contact information for a genetic counselor at a clinic in Chicago who had a lot of experience with the method. "Do me a favor, if you think you can," she told Amanda. "Contact them and listen to their explanation."

See concluded the talk by reminding Amanda of what it meant for her to have the GSS test. "This is a big decision," she said, looking Amanda in the eyes. "It will change the rest of your life. But if you go ahead, here is the procedure: when the results come in, you will go to your psychiatrist's office. The psychiatrist must be present and you will have to arrange for someone to drive you home afterward. Dr. Geschwind and I will call the psychiatrist's office and talk to you on a speakerphone. We will open a letter with your test results and read it to you—it will be the first time Dr. Geschwind and I will know what the test revealed. Then your psychiatrist will talk to you. Afterward, Dr. Geschwind and I will mail you a summary of the test data."

See would consult with Geschwind, she told Amanda and Brad, and tell him about their conversation. "Having the test will probably be one of the hardest things you will ever have to do, but I think you are prepared," she said.

"I hope so," Amanda replied. And then she and Brad left See's office in stunned silence.

There was no official routine for informing people about prion gene mutations. But Geschwind had seen enough families with prion diseases to be acutely aware of the pain of hearing the news, no matter how much people say they are prepared for it.

Leaving See's office, Amanda realized too that it had been one thing for her to say she wanted to be tested; it had been another thing entirely to spend an hour discussing what those results could mean. And the way she would be told—such a serious protocol, so different from the way her father and Uncle Billy had found out. Neither of them had been with a psychiatrist. Neither had spent time with a genetic counselor. The talk with See had been jarring, a blunt reminder of what was at stake.

"I'm doing the right thing," Amanda told herself. "Whether I am positive or negative I will be able to help with the research." She clung to that thought, numb and shocked by the morning she had been through.

The tests for Geschwind's study came next, standard cognitive tests, exactly like the ones her father had taken, also administered by Geschwind's staff. This included a mini-mental test that measures dementia: What city are you in? Who is the president? What year is it? She was also shown drawings, like a house or a cat, and asked what they represented. There were tests of her judgment: What would your response be if you saw someone breaking the law? And, as her father had done, she had to walk up and down the hallway as fast as she could. The tests were not hard, but all Amanda could think about was her father, here in this building, struggling to speak, trying to walk.

Finally, Amanda went to the lab and bared her arm for the needle that would draw her blood and determine her fate. She would have only two more months of not particularly blissful ignorance before hearing the result.

Doctors in Geschwind's group would also perform a spinal tap, although this was for the study. Brad and Amanda went together to the small windowless exam room where her spinal fluid would be drawn. This would require putting a needle into her spinal column and letting some of the fluid that bathed her spinal column and brain drip out into a test tube. Geschwind was looking for levels of a brain protein, tau. The thought was that one of the early signs of prion disease was increased levels of tau in spinal fluid.

Two doctors walked in and told Amanda to lie on her side on a narrow exam table, exposing her lower back where they would insert the needle. Then one of them asked Brad to leave the room. Her voice sounds so breathy, Amanda thought. Kind of like Darth Vader, like her voice is coming through a tunnel.

Amanda turned and stared in horror at the doctors. While her back was turned, they had donned bright yellow total body protection suits. Their heads were hooded, their faces masked, their eyes protected with huge plastic goggles. Their hands were gloved, their feet covered by boots.

"Why do you have those suits on?" Amanda asked, fear rising in her throat. The doctors explained it was to protect themselves, just in case she had the GSS mutation, just in case her spinal fluid had prions, and just in case the disease could be transmitted.

It made her feel as if she were toxic. Amanda turned her face away from them, determined not to let them see her cry. She wept silently throughout the procedure.

The final test was an MRI of her brain. Amanda had never had an MRI, and she worried about claustrophobia as she lay on the narrow ramp that slid into the tunnel of the big white machine. The technician told her she had to lie very still and placed big earphones on her head to muffle the clanging sounds of the rotating magnets. Still she could hear them banging and hammering in a staccato rhythm throughout. But after the spinal tap, this hardly felt like a challenge.

Amanda and Brad returned home without discussing the issue weighing on both their minds. Maybe the trip to Africa would be the turning point, Amanda hoped. At least when it was over they would finally know if she harbored that brutal gene.

# 13

# A Foreign Land

Amanda pushed San Francisco out of her mind as she prepared for her trip to Zambia. She'd be there for more than a month, from January 31 to March 2, 2009, at a place so foreign she could not even picture it. In the days leading up to her trip to San Francisco, she'd hardly thought about Zambia. Now it was all she thought about. She'd barely traveled outside the country—save for a few visits with her family to time-shares in the Caribbean, the Bahamas, and Grand Cayman—and she had never traveled alone. GSS had done this to her, she realized. She would be a different person if her father did not have the disease, if her great-aunt Faye and her uncle Billy and her grandfather had not had it. She would have had a predictable small-town life, probably as a doctor, like her dad. Oddly, in this way, the disease was opening her world.

She spent weeks planning the trip—searching the Internet for information on Zambia and the city of Livingstone in the southern part of the country, near South Africa, where she'd be staying. It was named after Dr. David Livingstone, the Scottish missionary and explorer. Another explorer, Henry Morton Stanley, had come across Livingstone in 1871 and, seeing another European man, asked the famous question: "Dr. Livingstone, I presume?"

As she prepared for her trip to Livingstone, Amanda pored

over photos of Victoria Falls, which was close by. She read and reread the information from African Impact so often she practically had it memorized. She asked the group to put her in touch with another volunteer who'd be going. They recommended she talk with a Florida nurse named Gemi; as it turned out, she would become Amanda's closest colleague in Zambia.

No one in the Baxley family had ever done anything like what she was about to do: she was not only going to Africa, but she was going by herself. And there was also a difficult secret being kept with regard to the trip. Amanda had only told Brad and her family and a couple of close friends that she would get the result of her GSS test when she returned. To everyone else, she'd given the other reason she was going—the more benign truth—to honor her father. He'd always dreamed of traveling and volunteering his medical expertise in different countries.

Finally, it was time to leave. Jittery, Amanda set off on the twenty-seven-hour trip. She'd chosen the cheapest route, which was indirect to say the least—Charlotte to Nashville, for a quick visit with Brad, then Nashville to Detroit to Paris to Johannesburg, where she'd spend the night before flying to Livingstone. San Francisco, which had seemed so different from what she was used to, suddenly seemed tame.

Twenty-seven hours later, Amanda found herself peering out over a mat of gray clouds as the small plane to Livingstone began its descent. The plane dipped lower, piercing the clouds. Looking down, she was stunned by the land's beauty, a brilliant green, like the South Carolina grass after a rainy spring day. She saw rolling hills studded with leafy trees. She drew in her breath in delight. She'd expected dusty brown earth, a few scraggly trees. Nothing like this.

With a small bump, the plane hit the runway and taxied to

a halt beside a white building. This was the airport, with its single gate. Amanda stumbled out of the plane and drew her breath. The bright sun blinded her and the heat choked her. She had never felt anything like it. It got hot in South Carolina but nothing like this. This was a sweat-draining, intense but dry heat.

And then there was the odor. The Chinese novelist Ha Jin once said that every country has its own odor. America, he wrote, smells "very sweet, like chemicals or a kind of perfume. It makes you sick for a while." But Zambia's odor was like an elixir to Amanda, so distinctive she would instantly be brought back to her short time there whenever she smelled it again, a fragrance that she came to wish could be bottled so she could be assured she could carry her African memories home. It was an odd smell, complex and irreproducible, an odor that to Amanda was clean, but with an undertone of sweat. She loved it.

She entered the baking hot terminal and went through customs, which, to her surprise, took no time at all. There was no luggage carousel, just a battered and scuffed metal table. A man threw bags on the table for travelers to grab.

Amanda found her bag and hauled it to another steel table for a security guard to examine. With a broad grin, he went through her belongings. When he saw the bags of vacuum-packed clothes tidily tucked into the contours of the bag he burst out laughing. Amanda laughed too. What must they think of her?

There was only one place to sit in the terminal building, a backless bench. Exhausted from her long trip, Amanda hauled her bag there and sat down to wait for a bus to take her to the African Impact hostel. About ten other people showed up, crowding onto the bench. Soon she was squeezed into a tiny space at the end of the bench. She gave up, rose from the bench, and walked to an open area. Lying on the beige tiled floor, she put her head on her bag, and dozed.

An hour and a half later, a battered white bus from African Impact pulled up. As it rattled down the rutted and potholed road, banging and shaking, Amanda and everyone else grabbed the backs of the seats on front of them, trying not to tip over.

Finally, the bus let Amanda off at the hostel where she'd be living. After she parked her bags in the small bedroom—there were three bunk beds lined up in a row for Amanda and the four other women staying in the room—she stepped outside and took in the town. It was desperately poor, with thatched-roof houses made of mud and streets strewn with trash. She wandered over to an open-air market and stared at the bustle of people who seemed hardly to notice the naked babies and children underfoot, crawling and toddling among the dusty narrow streets.

The days quickly fell into a pattern. At six thirty in the morning, an African Impact employee would bang on a pan to wake the group up. The five young women in Amanda's room would take turns using the one bathroom. Then they would dress and go outside to the eating area, two long tables in an L shape. They would serve themselves from a buffet table. Breakfast was always the same: instant coffee; toast and jam; the Zambian staple, nshema, which reminded Amanda of grits; oranges; and imbe, a bright orange fruit that tasted like mango. Their assignments for the week—such as working in the hospice house or in the fields—were written on a dry-erase board in the eating area.

Amanda and her roommates kept their windows open at night, but nothing alleviated the heat. They got used to sleeping under mosquito nets. It almost never rained, but when it did, the shower would quickly end and the water would dry almost instantly, leaving behind a clean grassy smell.

The workday began at 8:00 a.m. A bus took the volunteers to

their jobs, brought them back at noon for lunch, and then took them back to work until 5:00 p.m. At night, before she scrambled into her bunk bed to sleep, Amanda liked to wander over to the common area and lie on her back on the cement floor, her head cushioned by a rolled-up towel. Many nights there would be five or six other volunteers there, lying on the cement, staring in silence at the clear star-filled sky.

Work, for Amanda, meant rotating between four jobs. She worked as a nurse at a hospice house, where most patients had tuberculosis or AIDS. She worked at a rural pediatric clinic, where she maintained medical charts and talked to parents about boiling water before drinking it and about wound care and safe sex. She worked as a home health nurse, where she walked around Livingstone, visiting people who were unable to get to clinics. Most of these patients had tuberculosis or malaria or were starving. Amanda was their main source of health care, acting more like a doctor than a nurse. Finally, she did manual labor, intense work in the unrelenting heat, brick making and farming, slicing fields with a machete, and even helping a family build a house.

Every day, she walked three miles to an Internet café and tried to log on, but the connection was so spotty she often had to give up. When she could get through and managed to reach Brad by Skype, she would blurt out tales of patients at the hospice who had pierced her heart. There was the six-month-old baby girl with HIV. Amanda had taken the tiny infant outside, cuddling her in the shade of the hospice's covered porch, carrying her out back where there was a flower garden. The baby died shortly before Amanda went home.

She told Brad about a boy named Kennedy with a narrow face and a quizzical look. He was about eight or nine years old and had cerebral palsy. He lived at the hospice because his parents had died and there was nowhere else for him to go.

"He is such a sweet boy, so sweet," Amanda told Brad. "I sit on the porch with him and take him for walks around the house. He can't really talk, but he laughs and laughs and laughs. He is such a happy kid."

Then there was Amanda's best friend there, a small, animated twenty-seven-year-old African man named Brave. She met him a few days after she arrived and immediately warmed to his broad grin. He was the medical project coordinator, and that day, after telling the group about the work they'd be doing, he looked at Amanda and said, "If you cut yourself with a pair of scissors, blood will drop on the floor. The blood that will run out of your body will be red. If I cut myself with a pair of scissors, blood will drop on the floor. The same color, the same blood—no difference."

Amanda stared at him, overcome with emotion in this strange country that had welcomed her with no hesitation.

She watched as Brave taught AIDS awareness through dance, a revelation to Amanda. The performances were so energizing; it taught her there are more ways to communicate and instruct than simply talking.

In the evenings, when work was done, Amanda got in the habit of hanging out with Brave and a group of local people. They'd talk or listen to music on a battery-powered radio.

The work was all-consuming, and after her first homesick week in Zambia, Amanda almost forgot her life in the States. She became so deeply involved in the exhausting, exhilarating experiences she was having, she hardly thought about Hartsville or her family or GSS. And when GSS did enter her mind, it was in a different way now. There are many sorrows in life, especially in Zambian life, but you can still be happy. A disease—even one as terrible as GSS—does not have to destroy your inner self.

One day, Amanda went to a tiny barren home to visit a

woman who needed care. The woman held out her left foot—the big toe was rotting, necrotic, the tissue dying because of an infection. She needed antibiotics, but Amanda didn't have anything to offer her because volunteers were not allowed to carry prescription drugs. Yet if her infection was not treated right away, it could spread and she could lose her leg. "You need to be seen by a doctor at the clinic," Amanda told her. The woman replied that it was a long walk to the clinic and she had not eaten for four days; she was just too weak to make it there on her own. All Amanda could do was give the woman Tylenol for her pain and tell her she would try to arrange transportation to the clinic. She left the house, unable to stop thinking of that woman's plight: an infection that should be easy to treat eating away at her flesh while she stayed in her little house, starving and growing weaker by the day. Amanda never saw the woman again.

At the hospice center the next week Amanda met a young man named Joseph who had Parkinson's disease. He used to be a professional soccer player, he told her, and mourned the days when he could run, he missed it so. Amanda reluctantly thought of her father. She'd been nourished by this break from her own worries, but Joseph looked so much like Buddy toward the start of GSS. The facial expression that never changed, the blank stare. The shuffling gait, loud swallowing, trembling hands. The obvious weight loss. It broke her heart.

That afternoon, she and another volunteer woke Kennedy, the young boy with cerebral palsy, from his Haldol-induced sleep and pushed his wheelchair to the porch so he could sit with Joseph. The two had become friends, although Kennedy could not speak. They played together with Kennedy's toy truck under the shade of the porch, Joseph with his trembling hands, Kennedy with his shaky limbs.

Amanda's chest heaved. "This is just so beautiful," she

thought to herself. She considered these two lives, both stricken by disease and heartache, but also joined by this unlikely friendship. She wished she could do more, wished she had basic medical supplies, wished she was a doctor.

But even people who saw doctors often got little help. When the house handyman went to the medical clinic for a bad cut on his right index finger he was given Tylenol for the pain and told he'd have to have the finger amputated. The man was distraught—if his finger was amputated he would not be able to use his hand while it healed and he'd lose his job.

Amanda asked to take a look at his finger, swollen to three times its normal size. His palm and the front of his hand also were red and swollen, she noticed. She knew that if this had happened to him in the States, doctors would have cleaned and bandaged the cut and given the man antibiotics to take for two weeks. He would have been fine—and amputation would have been out of the question. But this was Zambia, where antibiotics were scarce, and even if they are available, almost no one could afford them.

Amanda fetched the first-aid kit she'd brought from home, opened it, took out Betadine, an antiseptic used to clean skin, and swabbed the man's cut. She wrapped his finger in gauze and taped it. In her kit was also an antibiotic, doxycycline. It would not be the antibiotic of choice in the United States as it is not powerful enough for an infection so severe. Still, Amanda thought, it would be better for him to take something rather than nothing. The man could not stop thanking her, but she wondered if she'd really managed to do anything for him.

For the next few days, she sought out the man when she came back to the hostel for lunch. He held out his hand while she cleaned and rewrapped his finger. On the third day, after Amanda had replaced the gauze, the man bent his finger back and forth and said, "I know God sent you and I thank him. I was going to lose this finger but you saved it. I couldn't move it and now look . . . I called my wife last night and told her 'This white lady from America saved my finger. She is here to volunteer and she didn't have to care about this but she does, and she checks on it every day. She really cares, and now I won't have to have it cut off. God sent her to me.' I thank you. I really thank you."

As she went about her days, Amanda sometimes looked around and wondered if she could ever explain her experience to her friends and family—the little mud streets and thatched-roof houses, the heat and the dust and the poverty, the sicknesses. They'd never understand. Neither would she before she actually came here. Now, though, she marveled at how people in this part of the world lived, how they managed to survive and be happy and joyful in such dire circumstances.

Toward the end of her trip she went to nearby Victoria Falls. She heard the roar of the water long before she actually saw it, and something about the immensity of the sight touched her that day in a way nothing else had. She broke down crying at the intensity of her experience, thinking of the test result that was to come. Then she lifted her arms and looked up at the cloudless sky. "No matter what happens to me, this is life," she thought.

Amanda arrived home on a sunny day, hot for South Carolina but chilly for Africa. She was brown from her days in the sun and was not wearing makeup—she had not worn makeup for a month. Kathy was there to pick her up from the airport.

They drove through Hartsville. It was so familiar, Main Street with its little shops, the lake, the parks. And yet nothing felt the same. Africa had changed Amanda. The next day she wandered through the town. She ran into people she knew and automatically mouthed the pleasantries. "Hey. How are you? Good to see you." But behind her disguise of familiarity, she felt offended by the most innocuous remarks, even by the abundance in the stores. Wandering through a supermarket, she was overwhelmed by the excess—the piles of fresh fruits and vegetables, and the meats, row after row, case after case of chilled roasts and hamburgers, chicken and sausages. It was jarring—all the things people felt they had to have and the way the smallest incident could ruin someone's day.

Amanda had come to think of Livingstone as home and the people she worked with as her family. "Every single ounce of me wanted to stay," she told Kathy. "I remember how I felt when I first landed in Livingstone—I remember thinking to myself, 'Wow . . . this is really going to be such a long month.' But after just a couple of days, I felt so at home. I remember feeling as if I had finally found where I belonged. I had finally found my place in the world. The time passed so quickly and I really, really, really wish that I had planned to stay in Livingstone longer."

Over and over, small incidents sparked vivid memories. In Africa, she frequently had to do a rapid blood test for malaria by slicing the person's finger with a razor blade. When she returned to Hartsville and got a nursing job nearby, she was able to prick patients' fingers quickly and painlessly with a fingerstick device. This inevitably reminded her of both the rigor and intimacy of Africa. She kept her memories to herself. It was useless to try to explain and people would get tired of hearing her.

She did make an effort to explain to Brad how Africa had changed her. "I was letting my risk and this disease kind of take over who I was," she explained. "It had been in my mind all the time. But then I was in this place where people are dying at thirty years old from poverty, from hunger. And yet they are the genuinely happiest people I ever met. They didn't let something like a disease affect them so much that they changed the way they lived. They showed me I don't have to let this disease make me give up on life. This is a gift from whoever is up above. I don't know how I would have dealt with it if I hadn't gone to Africa."

But as the day approached when she would learn the result of her test for the GSS gene mutation, Amanda lost some of her resolve. She realized that, in Africa, she not only saw others triumphing over hardship, she was also out of her world enough to avoid thinking too deeply about the reality of her life.

# 14

# Revelation

Amanda tossed restlessly, unable to sleep, in her old bedroom at her parents' house overlooking the lake; she wondered what she had gotten herself into. The next morning, she and Kathy and Brad would be sitting together in her psychiatrist's office, and she would find out if she had the mutated gene. She had set the process in motion and it was going to play itself out; there was no turning back. Staying in her childhood home, it was impossible to forget Buddy, sleeping in the bedroom down the hall. By now he was unable to talk, unable to eat anything but the pureed food Kathy fed to him. And it was impossible for Amanda to ignore the fact that by getting the test she was defying her mother's wishes.

But Amanda was so healthy, so bursting with life, that she just could not imagine such a fate befalling her. And Kathy, even while telling herself to be prepared for the worst, had also managed to convince herself that Amanda did not have the mutated gene. She told herself she had made peace with Amanda's decision. "Yes or no," she said to herself, "it will be okay." But she was banking on it being no.

Morning finally came, the thin rays of the first sunlight entering Amanda's darkened room, birds starting to chirp outside. It was one of those perfect days in early spring, bright blue sky, slight breeze. What could go wrong? Kathy met her downstairs, looking drawn. She had not slept either, Amanda thought. A caregiver had already arrived to take care of Buddy while Kathy was away. Amanda hugged her father, her arms around his thin chest, and cried silently. She needed the comfort of his words, but they were gone.

Amanda and Kathy set out for the forty-five-minute drive to the psychiatrist in Columbia. They were silent, each lost in thought, trying to calm their fears. Finally, Kathy spoke. She went over the pros and cons of finding out if Amanda had the gene. And she told Amanda again that getting the test result now, with Buddy so ill, was really difficult for her.

Amanda understood, but it was too late to have this conversation. In a few hours she would know. Yes or no. A life interrupted midway or opening to a full future.

Brad was going to meet them in Columbia. He shared Amanda's worries but also her strong conviction that she would be spared, so much so that he'd planned to return to his work as an intern in Nashville immediately after hearing the test result. He needed time to drive eight hours from Nashville to Columbia and then get back to Nashville again.

Brad's schedule at Vanderbilt was intense—he got one day off for every seven to ten days in the hospital. The only way he could take a day and a half away was to work thirty hours straight, banking the time he needed to be with Amanda. Even then, his plans assumed the news at the psychiatrist's would be good so he could turn around and drive right back to Nashville. He'd made no contingency plans. He squelched any nagging doubts, realizing, with a sick sense of dread that he had to assume Amanda did not have the mutation. It was just too horrible to contemplate the other outcome and raised too many questions about what would happen next. Should he marry her? Would they have children? Better to assume the best.

When his thirty-hour shift finally ended, Brad strolled out

of the hospital, went home, and took a nap, instantly plunging into the deep sleep of an overtired intern. That night he set off for Columbia in the old champagne-colored Ford Taurus that had belonged to his grandmother. He drove all night, arriving at the psychiatrist's office with a couple of hours to spare. Bleary-eyed, he parked in front of the small gray house that was the psychiatrist's office, staring at the low gate and the black wrought-iron fence and homey front porch. It looked so inviting, such a neat, comfortable little house. In a couple of hours he would be inside that door, he would be sitting in David Downie's office. Brad did not know him, but Amanda had sought his counsel starting in her college years, when Buddy got that terrible letter saying he had the GSS mutation. Whichever way it went that day, Brad knew, nothing would ever be the same. Then he closed his eyes and fell asleep.

As Kathy drove up to Downie's office, she and Amanda spotted Brad's car immediately. Amanda hopped out, opened the Taurus door, and shook Brad awake. Then the three walked in silence up the steps to the porch, pulled open the door, and entered. Downie came in and led them down a short hall. He had blocked off a few hours for them, so he could take as much time as needed. They walked into his office with its fireplace, a few soft chairs, a love seat. Downie sat in his chair behind his desk. Amanda sat by herself on the sofa. The others sat on chairs in a circle around the psychiatrist. Kathy was praying. Brad, holding a Star of David in his hands, was praying too. "Are you ready?" Downie asked as the phone rang. Amanda chuckled nervously. "As ready as I can be."

Downie pressed the button putting the call on speakerphone. Geschwind said hello, explained again that he was going to open the envelope and read the results out loud, and that he would be seeing the results for the first time. Amanda waited, whirling with a surreal, out-of-body feeling.

There was a moment of silence as Amanda imagined Geschwind slitting open the envelope, taking out the paper that would reveal her fate.

Then he came back on the line.

"I'm sorry, Amanda," Geschwind said.

She had thought she was prepared, but now she knew. Nothing, absolutely nothing, could ever have prepared her to hear this news. Nothing.

Amanda screamed. Brad and Kathy rushed to embrace her, but she pushed them away, not wanting to be touched. "Leave the room, please leave the room," she pleaded.

Kathy sobbed as she ran out to the hallway. She had had no idea how those words of Geschwind's would hit her. "My baby," she thought. "How can I help my baby?"

Brad wept, saying nothing as he walked out, his head bowed.

Amanda sat on the sofa, paralyzed with terror, staring at the floor as tears coursed down her face. Then she heard a sob and looked up at Downie. He was crying too. Finally, he spoke.

"How are you feeling, what is going through your head right now?" he asked.

"I just want to know what I am supposed to do now," Amanda replied, her voice choking.

"Amanda," Downie said, "I can't imagine responding to this the way you are responding. I am not that strong a person. I know you are very strong. I see it in the way you are reacting. I also know there is a part of you that doesn't feel very strong, a part of you that is really hurting now. I want you to know you have to let it out."

Amanda wept as one emotion after another washed over her—terror, despair, resolve, and terror again.

"I can't go there right now," she told Downie. "If I do, I will never come back. I can't parse where I am."

She lifted her head and looked straight at Downie, seeing

the tears that were continuing to roll down his face. Neither could speak. Then she gathered her courage and said her mother and Brad could return.

With trepidation, they entered the office.

"Okay. Okay," Amanda said to them. "Now what are we going to do about this?"

No one had an answer.

"I can't leave now," Brad thought. "I can't go back to Vanderbilt." But someone had to cover for him. He called his brother Ryan, also an intern, asking him through his sobs to help. Of course, Ryan said, of course he would cover for Brad. Then, forcing himself to sound calm, Brad called the chief resident at the hospital and explained that he had some personal problems. She allowed him to take more time.

Brad climbed into his car, numb, stunned, weeping silently as he followed Kathy and Amanda back to Hartsville.

When they arrived at the house, Kathy walked into the den where Buddy was reclining in his chair. She walked over to him and did something that she questioned then and ever after. She told Buddy. He looked at her and began to cry.

No one said much after that. Brad, Amanda, and Kathy wept; they hugged each other. That night, Brad went to Luke's room and Amanda went to hers. Because Brad and Amanda were not married, Kathy and Buddy did not allow them to stay in the same room in their house. Before Brad could even attempt to fall asleep, he heard a tapping on the door. It was Amanda. She nudged the door open and crept in. Brad held her close as they talked through the night about how unfair it all was and how it didn't seem real. They finally fell asleep, curled together in Luke's room, offering each other what scant comfort they could.

Brad had put off telling Amanda what he had to do next— he had to tell his parents. He had to go to Charleston to tell them in person. And he wanted Amanda to accompany him. He was sure she'd object. She knew his parents, his mother in particular, had always opposed the match. Yet when Brad asked Amanda to come to Charleston with him, she nodded numbly in agreement, beyond caring at this point what she did.

Although he did not tell Amanda, Brad had another reason for going to Charleston and for insisting Amanda come with him. He had been planning for some time to ask her to marry him and had bought a diamond, which he was storing at a jewelry store owned by his cousins while he saved up for a ring. The news about her gene test made him push up his schedule. It did not make sense any more to wait until he had an actual diamond ring to present to her. He had to ask her now so she would know he would stay with her. It was inconceivable to him to abandon Amanda now.

When Brad and Amanda entered his parents' house, he wasted no time getting to the point of their visit. After all, they knew Amanda was going to get her test results and, seeing his stricken face, it was clear that something terrible had happened. So Brad blurted out the news, watching as his parents' faces registered shock and sorrow. Then, as soon as he could, Brad took his mother aside. "I need your help," he said. "I want to pick up the diamond." He told Amanda he'd be back soon and drove off with his mother in her car. Amanda did not protest, did not even really question Brad. She wandered off by herself, lost in sorrow and terror.

Brad's mother told Brad she'd help—how could she turn down her son at a time like this? When they arrived at the jewelry store, he got out of the car and sat down on the curb, weeping. "I can't go inside," he sobbed. "I can't break down in front of them."

"That's okay, Brad. I will do it," his mother said. A few minutes later she was back, carrying a small baby blue box.

Inside was the diamond, carefully nestled in a square of crackly tissue paper. Brad did not say much on the drive back to his parents' house, and his mother kept quiet about her trepidation. When they arrived, Amanda was waiting, with that stunned look on her face, tear tracks on her cheeks.

"Let's go across the street to the field," Brad told her. It was their special place, suffused with happy memories. When both were living in Charleston—she in college, he in medical school—they used to take Brad's two Shetland dogs, Wrigley and Kady, to the field and play with them. That day, they got the dogs and threw a ball to them for a while. But Amanda was confused. Brad was acting strange, looking nervous. He was visibly shaking. After a few minutes he turned and faced Amanda and took out the little box.

"I wasn't planning on doing this today," he said. "So all I have is a loose diamond. But I want to be with you until the end. Will you marry me?"

## 15

# Of Two Minds

Amanda had kept the card that Patricia See had handed her with the name of a genetic counselor experienced with preimplantation genetic diagnosis. And she still remembered what See had said: "Do me a favor, if you think you can. Contact them and listen to their explanation."

At the time, it had all seemed so hypothetical. She had convinced herself she did not have the mutation and since she did not have it, she did not have to worry about PGD. Everything was different now. But she just was not sure she could go through with the procedure. Could she really agree to have embryos with the GSS mutation discarded like so much detritus?

Now that she knew she would be marrying Brad, her terror at the thought that she would get GSS was mingled with repeated thoughts of PGD. She and Brad talked about the procedure day after day, week after week. Brad was for it; he always had been. But Amanda remained opposed. She kept putting off what she knew she needed to do—call the counselor at the Chicago clinic. "A part of me is scared," she confessed to Brad.

She kept mulling it over as she adjusted to her new life with Brad. So much had happened in a blur after Brad gave her that diamond in the field near his parents' house. They rented a

U-Haul truck, packed all her possessions into it, and then drove to Nashville. They stuffed her clothes and books and CDs into the cramped room Brad was renting in a two-bedroom apartment and stayed there for a month of misery while they looked for a bigger apartment. Amanda found a job as a nurse at the Vanderbilt Stallworth Rehabilitation Hospital, helping patients with spinal cord and other traumatic injuries, a physically exhausting job that involved lifting and moving patients who were immobile.

GSS was always there at the edge of her consciousness no matter what she was doing or where she went.

In July, Amanda and Kathy went to Washington for a meeting sponsored by the CJD Foundation for families and patients with prion diseases. They'd discovered the group through the Internet. It was an advocacy group that raised money for prion disease research, and it helped families with prion diseases find each other and offered support. Brad and Luke wanted to go but could not get away from their work.

Amanda's older sister, Holly, preferred not to attend. She had taken the opposite approach, forcing herself to put her own risk of GSS out of her mind almost from the moment her father learned he had the illness. She decided not to be tested for the GSS gene. What would the test accomplish? It's not as though there was a way of preventing the disease or treating it. If she turned out to have the gene, all she would gain was the certainty that GSS would strike her. It would force her to live with a sword over her head.

"That is not the way I want to live as a Christian," Holly explained to her family. "It is not for me to know my future. That is in God's hands. God has a purpose in not creating us with the ability to know our end. I choose to trust Him." She worried privately that, as she saw it, "in a medical family, science often becomes god instead of God."

Holly was married and had a son when she learned her father had GSS, but she and her husband decided that Holly's risk of getting ill herself and of passing on the gene was not going to deter them from having more children. Soon after, she got pregnant and gave birth to another son. The looming GSS threat was not Holly's focus; she would not let it be. She saw getting past her fears and her desire to control her fate as a test of her faith. Instead of dwelling on the uncertainty of GSS, she would concentrate on her children's relationship with God, on their eternal life. "Hope and knowledge are mutually exclusive in this situation," she declared with fixed certainty. "While I don't know, I have hope."

Holly was all too aware that many, probably most, in her family would not make this choice. As time passed, she and others in her family dealt with their differences by seldom discussing their decisions about testing. To Holly, her family's reaction to the GSS threat often seemed overly emotional, even reflecting a lack of faith in God's plan.

Luke understood and even envied Holly's unwavering trust in God, but his faith was not that strong. For him, the dread of GSS was too real to ignore. His way of dealing with it was to learn all he could about the disease. For as long as he could remember he had wanted to be a doctor, but now he worried obsessively about what might lie ahead for him.

So with Holly keeping her distance and Brad and Luke unable to get away, it was just Amanda and Kathy who walked timidly into the meeting room on a steamy July day in 2009, a generic ballroom in a large Washington hotel, just down the street from the Capitol. Small round tables dotted the room, each with a pitcher of water and a small bowl of candy. They could have been in any city. They sat at a table in the very back, against the wall, wanting to be invisible.

Amanda had wanted to find out more about GSS and what research was being done and to talk to people like herself. But she was overwhelmed. She just was not prepared for this roomful of people each of whom had a spouse or a family member with a prion disease. Many had been tested for a mutated prion gene; some had discovered they had it and in some the disease had begun to take hold. Weeping, often sobbing, Amanda told people at the meeting that she too had inherited a GSS gene. "I'm sorry," they would say, always with a look of shock, always with tears.

But going to that meeting also was a turning point for Amanda. She met people who knew exactly what she was facing. She met researchers and the administrators of the foundation who said they would welcome her help talking to families who were as overcome as she was by the nightmare they had been thrust into. She felt a sense of purpose—she would do whatever she could to help the researchers and other families.

She also got to know Michael Geschwind better than she had during her visit to San Francisco. She watched as he patiently explained prion diseases to confused families, answering the same questions over and over with gentle concern and compassion. It struck her that for Geschwind, caring for people with prion diseases and studying prion diseases was more than a profession. It was a calling.

Amanda had hoped the scientific sessions would offer the promise of a cure or at least a treatment on the horizon, but that was not to be. Instead, researchers described what seemed like tiny steps and dashed hopes. The researchers were all too aware of the sense of urgency their audience had, their frustration with waiting while science took its careful and deliberate course, but with meager funds and little interest from funding agencies, they often found themselves stymied.

After that meeting, Amanda returned to Nashville and Brad, still wondering what to do about PGD.

Finally, she e-mailed the Chicago clinic and set up a time to talk. She was alone in the bedroom of their apartment, looking out at the quiet street below, when the counselor called her back. Her heart pounding, Amanda tried to pay close attention. The counselor told Amanda what would be involved if she had PGD, how couples feel about it, why they decide to do it. It would start with the onerous and emotionally difficult process of in vitro fertilization, with the added issue of testing and destroying embryos. Whether or not they believe life begins at conception, few can see a human embryo as just a clump of cells, no different in kind than a piece of skin scraped off a knee. And no one—not even people who work in fertility clinics where occasionally destroying embryos is part of the job—finds it easy to discard those balls of cells. Is it abortion? A medical abortion occurs after a pregnancy has occurred, which means an embryo has burrowed into a woman's uterus and started to grow. Is it morally the same? Amanda asked herself. That is where her agonizing began.

After an hour on the phone with the counselor, Amanda hung up, her eyes unfocused, feeling dazed. She wandered to the living room of their apartment, restlessly turning over the arguments.

Was she really willing to destroy embryos with the GSS mutation? If Kathy had had PGD, Amanda would never have been born. But if she could know for sure that one embryo had the mutation and the other did not, and if she had to choose just one, wouldn't she want the one without the GSS gene? It was not really a Sophie's choice type of situation. Still, half of her embryos on average would be killed. And because prion diseases were so rare and PGD so seldom used, no one had ever used this method to eliminate embryos with a prion gene mutation. She would be making medical history. Wasn't the first person to try something new taking a risk? The PGD experts would say it was no riskier than PGD for any other disease, but of course she had to assume they knew exactly how to test for that mutated gene in an embryo—it would require a custom-made test to look for her exact mutation in her prion gene—and she had to trust that there would be no lab errors, no careless mistakes.

She wavered, remembering all the times Brad had argued with her about PGD. He wondered whether it really was so awful to discard an embryo that was just a few days old, if those cells carried the GSS gene. Wouldn't Amanda want her own children? He certainly did, and this was a way—if she turned out to have the gene. He wanted to see his face and Amanda's in their children's faces, wanted her sparkly nature to shine in his kids, wanted to know his genes and hers were passed on and mingled in unpredictable but wonderful ways.

"I'm totally against it," she had told Brad every time he brought it up. But now, thinking of how much she wanted babies, how much she wanted to save her children from inheriting the GSS gene, she was altering her view. Maybe she could accept destroying embryos—still microscopic balls of cells— if she knew they had the dreaded gene. If she could be sure that her children would not suffer the fate that awaited her, why wouldn't she make that happen?

She had told Kathy about the procedure and at first, not realizing embryos would be destroyed, Kathy was overjoyed. "Oh, honey, that's wonderful," she exclaimed. Then she realized what would happen and quickly changed her mind, telling Amanda she could never give PGD her blessing. Amanda also told Luke, who thought it was a good option.

Ultimately Amanda was on her own, with a decision that she could talk herself into or out of from moment to moment. That day after talking to the counselor she finally decided. The answer was yes, she would do it.

Brad arrived home at his usual time, around seven, and, as he always did, methodically removed his jacket, his tie, and his shoes. Then he sat down on the sofa in the living room. Amanda sat next to him, turned, and held his gaze as her words flew out in a rush.

"I called the counselor in Chicago today. Brad, I think you are right about PGD. I think this is the way we have to go. I think we have to try it."

Brad hesitated. "Let's wait until we look at a printout of everything she said," he replied.

Amanda handed him a pamphlet. The counselor had e-mailed it to her and she had printed it. Side by side, she and Brad started to read.

Near the end they came to a breakdown of the cost—for medications, blood draws, ultrasounds, IVF, PGD: $22,000. Amanda looked at Brad, who was nervously flipping over the pages of the printout and reaching for a pen to start calculating.

"We knew it was going to be expensive," she said. "We had been told it would be expensive."

"Yes," Brad said, writing down each charge. "But we had absolutely no idea it would cost as much as this."

But Amanda had made up her mind. She was going to do everything in her power to avoid passing on the GSS gene to another generation. Even if it cost $22,000 to do so.

# 16

# A Unique Way

PGD was born out of decades of controversy in a medical field with a fraught history, eventually pushing it to the fringes of medicine, denied funding, and left to the private sector.

The tone was set in the 1960s, when a flamboyant British scientist, Robert Edwards, announced he was going to fertilize a human egg in a petri dish, grow it into an early embryo, and implant it in a woman's uterus. This, he declared, would ultimately enable many infertile women to have babies. If their fallopian tubes were blocked, for example, which was a common cause of infertility, sperm could not meet egg in the usual environment. The embryo could not start to develop as it floated down the fallopian tube to the uterus. He could bypass that step by starting a pregnancy in the lab.

Immediately, he was lashed with criticism. This was immoral and unnatural medicine, doctors objected. What made him think this practice would be safe? If he managed to fertilize an egg outside the body and then actually succeeded in creating a pregnancy, the baby more than likely would have birth defects or mental problems, critics charged.

The hostility drove Edwards, an embryologist, and his obstetrician colleague, Patrick Steptoe, underground. For nine years, Edwards traveled several times a week from his academic office in Cambridge to a little hospital in Oldham, England—a three- to four-hour trip each way—where he worked in secret in a tiny windowless lab.

The basic notion was straightforward, at least to Edwards. He wanted to mimic in a laboratory what normally happens inside a woman's body at the start of pregnancy. The process begins when, as happens every month, an egg matures and bursts out of the woman's ovary into her fallopian tube. There it meets with sperm, is fertilized, and starts to divide. The early embryo then floats down the tube to the woman's uterus where it burrows into the spongy uterine lining and starts to grow.

Edwards's plan was to remove mature eggs from a woman's ovaries before they could start their path down her fallopian tube. To fertilize them, he would mix them with human sperm in a petri dish. Then he would put the fertilized eggs in an incubator for several days, allowing the embryos to divide a few times and grow. Many would die at that point, he realized, partly due to the unnatural environment and partly because, even in a natural pregnancy, many eggs that are fertilized in a woman's fallopian tube die before a pregnancy can be established.

Edwards would use the fertilized eggs that had survived, turning into early human embryos, to try to initiate a pregnancy by placing them in the womb of an infertile woman. There, hopefully, they would survive and grow, developing into a fetus and ultimately a baby.

In practice, however, every step of the procedure presented difficulties. Finding a source of human eggs was hard enough. Edwards began asking gynecologists if they would give him slices of ovaries they had removed for medical reasons. Most scoffed, telling him it was a preposterous idea. But, finally one doctor, Molly Rose, who had delivered two of Edwards's five daughters, agreed to do it.

But the eggs in those slices of ovaries were immature and

immature eggs cannot be fertilized. That meant the researchers had to figure out a way to make the immature eggs buried in those ovaries ripen until they were ready to be fertilized. It took the scientists two years to achieve this goal. In 1972, they succeeded. Edwards wrote of his "joy unbounding" with this achievement.

Then they had to find a way to prompt sperm to fertilize these eggs. It took two years before they could bring this step to fruition. Next, they had to get the fertilized eggs to grow in their lab. And, finally, they were ready to attempt the most difficult task of all: achieving a pregnancy in a woman.

Over the course of several years, Edwards and Steptoe tried more than a hundred times with patient after patient before they finally achieved this goal. In 1977, they managed to get through every step successfully with a British woman, Lesley Brown, who had previously tried for nine years on her own to become pregnant.

The two doctors trumpeted their success.

On July 26, 1978, Brown was ready to give birth and the press descended en masse on the small hospital in Oldham where she had been admitted. Edwards left the hospital that afternoon and told the crowd of reporters and onlookers that nothing was happening yet and they could go home. He and Steptoe snuck in the back entrance that night and Steptoe delivered the baby by cesarean. This had nothing to do with medical necessity; Steptoe and Edwards wanted to control when and where the baby was born so they could avoid having reporters lurking outside the delivery room. If the baby had been abnormal, that would have spelled the end of IVF.

Fortunately, the baby, Louise Brown, was healthy—and an IVF industry was born. But the initial hostility and suspicion about the procedure set the pitch for what was to come. Though in 2010 Robert Edwards would be awarded a Nobel Prize for his fertility work, at this time in the United States, the federal government refused to pay for research on human embryos, so the work was done in private clinics that wanted to make a profit selling the procedure. In a few states, like Illinois, it was illegal for years for anyone—including doctors in private clinics—to practice IVF.

From the start, IVF had problems: women miscarried, they had triplets, quadruplets and more. If their babies were born alive, they were sometimes born weeks or months premature and spent long periods in intensive care, often ending up with brain damage or blind or deaf or with cerebral palsy. Drugs women were taking to produce multiple mature eggs for the procedure were causing some to experience a dangerous condition—hyperstimulation of the ovaries, which made ovaries grow as big as grapefruits. And the overall results weren't promising: pregnancy rates were as low as 10 percent at the start.

Gradually, fertility doctors figured out how to improve IVF; now they have pregnancy rates of 70 to 80 percent within two to three IVF cycles in healthy women younger than age thirty-five and rarely have the complications that plagued the early days.

More than a decade after the first IVF birth, while the method was still ineffective, a second wave of controversy arose. Several groups, including one led by a flamboyant Russian geneticist and embryologist, Yury Verlinsky, decided it was time to take another bold step: preimplantation genetic diagnosis. Doctors would start the IVF process, but while the embryo was still just a tiny cluster of cells, they would pluck out a cell or two and analyze it for genetic defects.

PGD had been successful in animals, but it had never been attempted with a human embryo. So before he began, Verlinsky called a group of experts together to discuss whether it would work in humans. They met at Chicago's Drake Hotel in September 1990. Most of the attendees were lab scientists, PhDs. But one of the few fertility doctors there, James Grifo of New York University, had experience in both realms—IVF in humans and PGD in animal studies. He came to present the data from his studies with mice, reasoning that because the method had worked in animals it would work in humans. "It's pretty much true that anything that works in animal systems seems to hold true in humans," he said. Bob Edwards came, too, speaking at length about PGD and what it might mean to couples.

For all their bravado, however, it took nearly a decade before PGD was ready for even the most narrow use—and then the number of conditions it could test for was extremely limited. Only a few medical centers dared try it and those that did sometimes made mistakes, proclaiming embryos free of a gene mutation when actually they were not. The testing in those days was for fatal or debilitating diseases that arise in infancy or childhood, so when mistakes were made, they were obvious. The error rate was as high as 5 percent. There was anguish, heartache and lawsuits.

Verlinsky's group was among those trying PGD, but it was having the same difficulties as everyone else: most women did not get pregnant and the lab sometimes made errors. Then Verlinsky asked a talented Israeli fertility doctor, Ilan Tur-Kaspa, to come to Chicago and work with him. Tur-Kaspa was an expert at IVF, and his work at Verlinsky's institute got off to a stunning start—of the first ten women who came to Tur-Kaspa for IVF with PGD, eight became pregnant, an unheard-of rate even today.

Verlinsky was ecstatic. But Tur-Kaspa injected a note of caution. "The only thing I can guarantee you is that the pregnancy rate will go down," he warned. Of course it did—the initial result was a statistical fluke.

But Tur-Kaspa's reputation was made. Now Verlinsky's institute, already well known for its expertise and bravado, had become a mecca for those seeking PGD.

Eventually the method became more foolproof. The result today is a 1 to 2 percent error rate in the ten thousand embryo tests Verlinsky's center performs each year, mostly embryos sent from medical centers around the world for genetic analysis. Other centers that do PGD have similar results.

But the method is not without critics. It has been used to eliminate embryos with gene mutations for diseases, like breast cancer, that make the condition more likely but not inevitable. And it has been used to eliminate embryos with genes for diseases, like GSS or cancer or an inherited form of Alzheimer's disease, that do not occur until midlife or later. Does that mean that people with those gene mutations should never have been born?

Its defenders often point to the diseases that strike infants or babies, killing them when they have barely had a chance to live. Those of course are the easiest cases. But they also say it is not for them to judge, which some might view as ducking the issue.

"Imagine having your baby die of a disease and knowing there is a 25 or 50 percent chance the next baby will have those problems," Grifo, the fertility doctor at New York University, explains. "Talk to a patient first before you judge. I have learned the most amazing things about human beings by listening to people talk. People can live through and withstand the most amazing things and turn it into something good. We figure out a way for them to have the family they want. That is huge."

Tur-Kaspa shares his sentiments. "The way I look at it is, you are the patient. You carry the genetic disease." Studies, he said, have shown that most patients do not want donor eggs or sperm. Nor do they want to adopt. And most do not want to conceive on their own, a process Tur-Kaspa calls reproductive roulette—only to have an abortion if the fetus is affected. The way he sees it, IVF with PGD is giving patients incredible options. After years of doing IVF with PGD, Tur-Kaspa says he has seen what seems like every variation of human turmoil over genetic diseases. And he has learned to keep an open mind as a result.

But with scientists' increasing ability to find genes that increase risks for disease, the questions might get more difficult. Suppose, for example, a man has a gene that gives him a 50 percent chance of having a heart attack by age fifty-five. Should he and his wife eliminate that gene with PGD?

For now, though, many of those questions are hypothetical. Most common disorders—obesity, autism, low intelligence—are not linked to a single gene. Instead, hundreds of genes seem to be involved. It may not be so simple to engineer the ideal human being.

Tur-Kaspa, for one, urges critics who fear the ethicists' slippery slope to focus on what is possible now.

"Right now, do I have to answer yes or no to every theoretical model?" he asks.

But Tur-Kaspa is certain of one thing: "This is a unique way to bring a child into the world."

## 17

# "We Have No Other Options"

"We can do this."

Brad went through his list of calculations. They had savings, about $8,000, but their incomes were paltry. He was still in medical training as a resident at Vanderbilt University and was taking home about $38,000 a year—$3,100 a month—while working eighty hours a week. And Amanda, he pointed out, was working three twelve-hour shifts a week, and making about the same amount.

But if he moonlighted, Brad exclaimed, his eyes bright with enthusiasm, if he took on extra shifts, he could accumulate an extra twenty hours a week at $150 an hour. That would nearly double his salary. Amanda chimed in—she could volunteer for extra nursing shifts. And she had an offer from a family who wanted to hire her to babysit ten hours a day on her days off. That would bring in an extra couple of thousand a month.

They looked at each other, smiling nervously; they were daunted by the commitment but ready to take it on. Their combined efforts, with nonstop work, could bring in nearly $5,000 in extra cash each month.

Brad pointed at their list of expenses. The biggest savings, he said, would come from finding a cheaper apartment—they were currently paying $1,200 a month. The deprivation of a smaller apartment would be temporary and they had to get started with PGD fast. It might not work the first time, after all, and Amanda was twenty-seven. Even at Amanda's age—still several years before her fertility would start to decline—for every hundred women trying to have a baby with IVF, forty to fifty fail on the first attempt and have to try again another month. And then, of course, there was GSS, looming as ever. The longer they waited to try to have babies the less time she would have with her children before the illness would take over.

They'd ruled out using their health insurance, which sometimes will pay for at least part of the procedure. They wanted to keep the knowledge of Amanda's GSS gene to themselves. The laws that prevent employers from discriminating against people with genetic disorders would not go into effect until November of that year. As for health insurance, this was before the Affordable Care Act of 2014, which prevents insurers from discriminating against people with preexisting conditions. Amanda faced the risk of being denied employment or health insurance if she changed jobs. And there still isn't a law prohibiting life insurance companies or long-term care insurers from denying coverage to people with gene mutations.

They never considered asking Brad's parents or Kathy to pay for the procedure, never even discussed that as an option. Both instinctively assumed the bill was their responsibility.

It was also understood that, although Kathy was proud of Brad and Amanda for taking on the burden of PGD, she would never pay for a procedure she felt was morally wrong.

So they began.

Brad immediately got lucky in his apartment search, finding a newly built complex geared toward college students and young professionals. The rent would save them $300 a month. Amanda went to take a look on her day off, a cold gray winter morning. She gazed up at the three-story brick building on a noisy, busy street. But she saw a park nearby, and a grocery store. She wandered around the exterior. The apartments were built around a courtyard with grass and a few trees and a pool. The apartment itself was tiny, unfortunately, about the size of a room in an extended-stay hotel. Amanda made a video of the place and showed it to Brad that night. They talked themselves into it. It was the best they could do for the money. They took it.

Amanda felt so clever as she planned how to make that apartment livable. Too many clothes and not enough closet space? She bought risers for the bed and stashed nonessential clothes underneath. She bought a rolling rack, like the ones used by dry cleaners, to hang clothes they wore every day.

No room to store cans and dry goods and boxes? Amanda went to Target and bought shelving. Later, when she visited, Kathy sewed curtains to cover the shelves.

Meanwhile there was work—endless work—to make that extra money. The days and weeks became indistinguishable; Amanda and Brad were constantly exhausted, but their ruthless pursuit of their goal carried them along. Simple things—shared naps on rare days when they were both at home or lunches together at the hospital—took on the sweetness of stolen time.

Brad soldiered on pragmatically, refusing to be plagued by thoughts of what was at stake. He never voiced doubts about their decision to use PGD. But nagging worries crept into Amanda's thoughts. What if they went through all this sacrifice and the procedure didn't even work? And if it did work, how could she justify bringing children into the world only to have them watch her suffer and die?

The constant work, life in that tiny apartment, the uncertainty, the stress, began taking a toll. Despite their resolve not to let their circumstances diminish their love, there were times when they would snap at each other, times when their anxiety and exhaustion led them to say things they immediately wished they could take back.

And the fact that her mother did not approve of the PGD procedure made Amanda feel that much more alone. The testing center wanted a swab of cells from Buddy's cheek so they could make sure that Amanda and Buddy had the same mutation. Buddy was too ill by then to communicate, but Kathy knew he would disapprove of PGD as strongly as she did; she knew that he would refuse the cheek swab. The answer was no. It was agonizing for Kathy to deny her child, and Amanda was furious, refusing to talk to Kathy for two weeks. But Kathy was haunted by the idea that if she herself had had PGD—if she had known about GSS and that Buddy had the gene—she would have discarded the embryo that became Amanda.

Holly felt PGD was unnatural, even sinister. "That idea carries with it the potential to create a medically induced genocide with the murdering of preborn children as a way of manipulating the gene pool and producing a utopia," she said. "Humans with too much knowledge are dangerous."

Kathy made her views explicit to Amanda, talking them through, whereas Holly preferred to avoid the subjects of GSS and PGD altogether.

But Amanda did have Luke, as always. He wholeheartedly approved of PGD. Though he had never heard of it until Amanda told him about it, he said that if he had the gene he would want to use this method too.

Once, in a moment of intense doubt, Amanda asked Brad how he was so sure about their decision. "We have no other options," Brad said firmly. "This is something we have to do and we will get through it." They were in it too deeply now to back away.

★ ★ ★

When Amanda turned from the thorny issues of PGD, she often found herself facing another problem: she and Brad both wanted to have a wedding, but the question of where to hold the wedding was proving impossible to answer. The dilemma involved Buddy—he was extremely ill now, miserable with muscle spasms so severe that his entire body contracted. Sitting in his wheelchair, he'd stoically endure excruciating cramps, his body tense, his foot jiggling. He was starting to choke on his own saliva. He could not eat without coughing and sputtering. He could not drink. Often he did not recognize people now, even his own family, including Kathy. He could not speak, nor could he use the alphabet board to communicate any longer.

Amanda wanted to have the wedding elsewhere—a destination wedding—but also knew that this would exclude Buddy because travel was out of the question for him. The other option, of course, was a big southern wedding in Hartsville, with her father in attendance.

Kathy told Amanda she wanted Buddy to be present at the wedding, even if he disrupted it with loud spells of choking. Other relatives felt the same way. Uncle Mike. Uncle Tim. Her grandmother, Merle. They were unwavering in their disapproval of Amanda's desire to get married elsewhere. The wedding should be in Hartsville, they said, and Buddy should be there. Brad also wanted the wedding in South Carolina so that his elderly grandmother could attend.

Mike offered to pay for part of the wedding if Amanda had it in Hartsville. She refused. Tim called Kathy and told her that in his opinion a destination wedding was cruel. He and Mike both said they would not come if the wedding was held far from Hartsville and neither would Merle.

Amanda did not really expect Holly to come—she disapproved of so many of the circumstances in Amanda's life: the

PGD, her marriage to a Jewish man. And, beyond that, Holly refused to step foot on an airplane. Flying terrified her. She had flown once when she was eleven years old—when the family went on vacation in the Bahamas—and she never set foot on an airplane again.

So when Holly declined the invitation, Amanda was not surprised. But she was wounded by her uncles' reactions. Still, she winced every time she envisioned the scene if her father was there, in the church, at her wedding. He'd be in the front, a caregiver at his side. People would stare at him and then avert their eyes. Those who knew she had the gene mutation—family, close friends—would murmur behind cupped hands that Amanda would end up like that. They would feel sorry for Kathy and for Amanda; they would wonder whether it made Brad brave or foolish to marry into a family with that disease. A day that should be joyous would be sullied by the grim reminder of GSS—the dark cloud that had cast a shadow over her entire adult life.

"I honestly could not care less if he interrupted our wedding," Amanda told Brad. "But I know it would matter to him."

And yet Amanda privately wavered on this point. If her dad could speak, he would say he would never want to be the center of attention at her wedding. But the former Buddy, the Buddy before he had gotten so sick, would never have missed the ceremony. She didn't know which version of her father to honor.

The choice weighed on Amanda, tortured her, until, finally, she decided that her father would not want her to be so worried about it. She told Brad she had come to a decision. "Dad would say, 'This is your wedding. If you want to have it wherever, just do it. I will be there in my heart.'" Brad wondered, would Amanda feel she was giving in to GSS if she had the wedding in Hartsville? Having a destination wedding and being free was a gesture of defiance, a way for her to disown the disease a little bit, he told himself. This, he decided, was Amanda's decision; he would go along with whatever she wanted.

So they'd get married in Jamaica. She'd have it without her uncles Tim and Mike and their families in attendance. Without her grandmother Merle. But Luke would be there, of course. He and Amanda were so close; he would never miss her wedding.

Despite her continued internal questioning—Am I hurting my dad? Is this the wrong decision?—she told Kathy that her mind was made up. And Kathy, who would be paying for the wedding, struggled with her own conflicting emotions. How could Buddy be excluded, left at home while his youngest daughter celebrated in Jamaica?

But Kathy always believed that she should not manage her children's lives. They were adults and had to find their own way, and although she could tell them her opinions, she had to let them make their own decisions. She would go to Jamaica, where her daughter could escape GSS, if only for the day.

As the wedding day grew near, Amanda had an idea. After she and Brad returned from Jamaica, they could have another reception, at home in Hartsville. She would wear her wedding dress. She would dance. Buddy could come.

Amanda and Brad planned to have the wedding at a Sandals resort in Jamaica. They invited fifty guests—twenty-four accepted. The resort made it easy for them—its staff would provide the music, the flowers, the cake. It would be a melded Jewish-Christian ceremony, with Brad's uncle representing Brad's religion during the ceremony and a minister supplied by the resort representing Amanda's.

Kathy went to Buddy, slumped over in his chair, watching

television. She bent over and looked into his eyes. "Buddy," she said. "Amanda is getting married in Jamaica." He did not—could not—respond. But he stared at Kathy with those bulging eyes, and she had a sense that he heard her and realized he was being excluded from his daughter's wedding. Yet she had to tell him—how could she not?

Amanda and Brad's plane landed in Montego Bay on a bright sunny afternoon in January, two days before the wedding. Stepping off the plane, inhaling the unique Jamaica smell—sweet like flowers but also with a slight scent of charcoal—Amanda sighed and grinned. This was so far from the cold gray winter in Nashville. She and Brad climbed into the backseat of a battered taxi and held hands for what turned out to be a harrowing ninety-minute taxi ride to the hotel as the flimsy cab lurched over deeply potholed roads. The smiling and unflappable driver delighted them as he randomly stopped and picked fruit from the surrounding trees, presenting it to Brad and Amanda as a gift from his country. They had not expected that jarring taxi ride, but it was a good start, a charming introduction to Jamaica, if a bit rattling.

Amanda and Brad abandoned themselves to the moment, putting their dreary lives in Nashville behind them. They quickly pulled on their bathing suits and headed for the white sand beach. They swam in the lucid aqua water, they lay on padded lounge chairs in the hot sun, they sipped big tropical drinks on the veranda, they napped. Brad had struggled the entire trip to avoid falling asleep—he'd worked for thirty hours straight before boarding the plane—but now that he had arrived, he felt a burst of energy.

Two days passed in a sort of blissful haze. Yet Buddy was always on the edge of Amanda's consciousness. Would he understand why he was alone in that big house in Hartsville save for a caregiver? Did he feel abandoned? She tried to push those thoughts from her mind, but they remained always humming in the background, a troubling reminder that there was no real escape; this was an illusory departure from her life.

On the afternoon of their wedding, Amanda and Brad watched the staff prepare. Workers had stretched a long white carpet from a cluster of trees near the veranda down to the beach. At the end of the carpet, they set up a chuppah, a square white canopy held up with bamboo posts, traditional in Jewish weddings, symbolizing the home they would make together. It was another perfect day. The resort had planned the ceremony for the waning hours of the afternoon when the heat was starting to dissipate.

The wedding itself was a blur for Amanda, so high on the excitement of the moment she barely registered where she was or what she was doing. Kathy sang "How You Live," by the contemporary Christian group Point of Grace. Luke walked Amanda down the aisle. Amanda glanced at the guests as she approached the chuppah, a smile of sheer delight on her face. Brad, wearing a yarmulke, grinned nervously as she came down the aisle.

They had written their own vows and did not tell each other what they would say. But as they spoke, Amanda realized they had used the same website for inspiration and that some of the phrases they chose were identical. She burst out laughing during the ceremony when she heard their duplicate sentiments, realizing later that people must have wondered what was so funny.

When the brief ceremony came to an end, Brad, in keeping with Jewish tradition, stomped on a wine glass that had been wrapped in a cloth napkin. At last he and Amanda were married. Never had the words "in sickness and in health" meant so much.

They streamed the ceremony to Buddy back at home in Hartsville, who watched it in his wheelchair, Holly at his side.

Then Brad and Amanda and their guests went to the veranda where a DJ was playing Jamaican music. Everyone took their shoes off and danced. Waiters and waitresses joined in. Amanda and Brad forgot the fatigue that had dogged them in Nashville; they pushed their real lives out of their minds. They were so ready to have a good time, to let loose at last. They could worry about tomorrow when tomorrow came.

Four days later, Amanda and Brad got off the plane that returned them to Nashville. The tingly exhilaration that had buoyed them in Jamaica rushed out of them at once, like air from a deflating balloon. They flew to Hartsville the next week for a reception at a big white two-story building in a park near Buddy and Kathy's house. About 150 people came, some arriving in a chartered bus from Charleston. Buddy was there too, in his wheelchair, bent over and drooling, showing no sign he understood what was going on. But Amanda was glad to have held the reception with her father there—it was, she realized, more for him than for her.

Then it was back again to the tiny apartment. Back to the unending work. Back to the constant thoughts of GSS and PGD and what was in store for them. How could that magical time and their feelings of pure abandonment have come and gone so quickly? They went through what they thought of as a mourning period. Mourning for the fleeting happiness they had left behind in Jamaica.

Mourning for what they could never have—a normal life, a normal family, babies conceived the normal way.

But in less than a year they had saved half of the money they needed for PGD. They had set something in motion that would change their lives.

Two months later, Kathy called Amanda. Buddy was no longer able to eat or drink. "It's time," she told her daughter. Time to come home to see her father before he died.

Amanda got on a plane, arriving in Hartsville the next day. She spotted Kathy immediately when she went to the baggage claim area, looking gray and drawn as she hugged her daughter and led her to her car. They barely spoke as Kathy drove to the familiar house on the lake. Amanda walked into the hallway, dropped her bag, and went immediately to the back bedroom where her father was lying, mute and still, but awake. Hearing his daughter come into his room, Buddy turned his head and trained his eyes on her as she sat on the bed beside him. Amanda said nothing as she stared into her father's eyes. She and Buddy stayed that way, eyes locked, for half an hour. Amanda felt a powerful pull as if her father was trying to infuse her with strength for what lay ahead and also silently communicate to her that while he wanted her there, he also did not want his baby girl to see what had become of him.

Finally, Buddy closed his eyes. Amanda hugged him as she wept. She told him she loved him, told him how much he meant to her. He could not respond.

Luke, a resident in emergency medicine in Charleston, had arrived the day before. His job was to keep Buddy comfortable with intravenous morphine, providing more care than the hospice workers who had been coming could offer.

Holly visited on the weekends when she did not have to work. Despite tensions that had developed—about life decisions made, about how to handle GSS—the family now came together, almost as a team. Amanda and Kathy did the nursing, Luke was the doctor, and Holly made sure everyone was fed, the house was in order, and the laundry was done.

"If you have to die of this terrible disease, doing it this way is a gift," Kathy told her children. Buddy remained at home, he was kept comfortable, and even though he seemed less and less aware of his surroundings, his family was with him.

Finally, Amanda had to return to Nashville and to work. She did not want to leave and told Buddy so as she tearfully said good-bye, hugging and kissing her father and knowing it was probably for the last time. By then, Buddy no longer recognized her.

The next morning her phone rang. It was Kathy. "He's gone," she said.

Amanda returned to Hartsville that day and stayed for a week, helping Kathy, grieving with her mother, with Luke and Holly, with her uncles and her tiny grandmother, Merle, who had already seen her husband and oldest son die of this disease.

# 18

# Prescription Fertility

One morning a month after her father died, Amanda woke with a resolve. She and Brad had saved enough money. It was time to start a new life. It was time for promise to displace sorrow.

She picked up her cell phone and called the Reproductive Genetics Institute in Chicago. "I want to start PGD," she said. The first step, she was told, would be a phone consultation with the doctor, Ilan Tur-Kaspa. Amanda knew he was well-known, she knew the Chicago clinic had a good success rate, but she did not know just how experienced and pathbreaking Tur-Kaspa was in his field. He had performed more than a thousand PGD procedures and though he had never done PGD for a patient with a prion disease, the basic steps were the same. Start with in vitro fertilization, then let an embryologist pluck a few cells from the embryos that were starting to develop in petri dishes. A geneticist would test those cells for the GSS mutation and the lab staff would discard any embryos that had it. Tur-Kaspa would insert a healthy embryo into Amanda's uterus.

A week later Tur-Kaspa called. Amanda noticed his Israeli accent and pictured a solemn, middle-aged doctor, a bit heavy and very serious. He explained that for the IVF part, a pharmacy would send Amanda a sequence of medications that would prod her ovaries to overproduce eggs. The idea was to get as many eggs as possible to mature so they could be extracted from her ovaries and fertilized in the lab. That would give her the best chance of having at least a few healthy embryos without the GSS mutation.

Amanda would need to inject herself with these medications every day—as is routine with IVF—using a small sharp needle like those used by people with diabetes when they inject insulin, inserting the needle near her belly button. She'd start with a hormone that prevents ovulation until multiple eggs are ready as well as a hormone that stimulates the development of multiple eggs. Toward the end of the month she would inject a hormone that spurs the final maturation of the eggs. She'd have ultrasound exams every week or so to monitor the eggs' progress and the scans would be sent to Tur-Kaspa, who would oversee the procedure from his office in Chicago.

When her eggs were ready, Amanda would go to the institute in Chicago. There, Tur-Kaspa would extract the eggs by inserting a thin catheter into each egg-containing follicle and carefully removing them. Brad would be on hand to provide a sperm sample to fertilize the eggs. Fertilization would take place in a lab, under a microscope. An embryologist would inject a single sperm into each of her eggs.

It took a month before everything was in place and the first package of medications was due to arrive. Amanda had planned the delivery for her day off. She woke early, jittery with excitement and trepidation, waiting for the FedEx truck. She paced, looked out the window, went back and sat on her couch. Jumped up and looked out the window. Paced some more. Went back to the couch. Got up. She could not stay still.

Finally, in the early afternoon, the truck arrived and she got her package. Impatiently, she tore open the box and saw a big silver pouch and several smaller boxes. The pouch was filled with dry ice and little vials of Lupron, which would prevent ovulation until multiple eggs were ready. Nestled alongside it were syringes, alcohol wipes, and gauze pads, as well as other drugs, like progesterone suppositories to prepare her uterus, and Gonal-f, which would be used at the end of the month to stimulate ovarian follicles to release their eggs. One syringe—the one filled with Gonal-f—was so large it looked barbaric. Amanda shuddered.

She took the vial of Lupron out of her refrigerator and nervously attached a thin needle to its base. She rubbed ice over her belly to numb it. Then she hesitated, needle poised, unable to jab it in. She just could not do it. "I'm a nurse," she told herself. "I know how to give injections. I do it all the time."

She sensed that her skittishness over the injection was more than just simply fearing the needle's plunge into her skin. Once she began, once she started this process with that first injection, she was committed. She would have decided for certain that she was going to go all the way—to have IVF, to have PGD, to discard embryos with the mutation. She would bring children into the world who would escape her fate but who would have to watch her die the way she had seen her own father slowly robbed of himself. Seen her grandfather. Seen her uncle Billy. She looked down at the needle in her hand.

Yes, she told herself, this is what we want. This is why we live in this tiny apartment. This is why we work endless hours. She pushed the needle in. The deed was done.

The shot, it turned out, was nothing. But the medicine, the medicine burned going in. She gasped, her eyes stung with tears. She'd had no idea it would hurt like that. Somehow, the shock of that fiery medicine took her mind off the enormity of the process she had started. Later, though, the relentless thoughts came back. She had begun. But was it right?

Amanda hadn't counted on the side effects. They were as

big a surprise as the burning when she injected herself, but worse, much worse, for someone as conscious of her appearance as she. She'd always prided herself on being lean, athletic looking, and attractive, the sort of woman men noticed. She had always taken care with her hair, her makeup. She knew how to use eyeliner and mascara to make her eyes look huge and she was rarely without lipstick. Now, almost overnight, because of the progesterone, she gained fifteen pounds, which showed up in her abdomen, shoulders, and face. She stared at herself in the mirror. Unrecognizable, she decided. She looked so puffy— her eyes were narrowed, her cheeks bulged. She could not button her pants. This was not her.

"You look great," Brad told her. "You needed to put on weight anyway."

Kathy tried to console her. "Amanda, you know why you are doing this. The weight gain is a side effect. It will go away."

The hormones also affected her mood. She felt hot, tired, irritable. She tried to talk herself out of her peevishness. Remember your goal, she told herself. Don't let the drugs get to you. Don't focus so much on what you look like. Be grateful for Brad. You should be grateful to have this chance. But these internal pep talks were of little use. Cold logic was no match for her emotions.

And like every married couple, Amanda and Brad had their frictions, magnified by their harrowing lives. Nothing, it seemed, had ever been easy for them and sometimes it all seemed unbearable, saving money for PGD, living in that claustrophobic apartment. The prowling threat of GSS. Knowing they were trying to have children who would all too soon have to watch their mother sicken and die. Knowing Brad would have to be the caregiver. Sometimes it seemed like happiness was a promise they could never quite achieve.

Of course they argued. Blowups seemed to occur weekly,

if not more often. "What are we doing?" one of them would exclaim. Little things would flare into major disputes. Amanda would dash out of the apartment, slamming the door, driving away and not returning for several hours while she and Brad fumed.

But they stayed together, bound by their love and their fervent desire to have children, their own children. And they wanted children who did not have the gene for GSS, who would be spared the struggle and the worries they were going through.

Once a week, on one of her days off, Amanda went to the imaging center for an ultrasound to monitor the size of her ovaries. The place was always filled with pregnant women. Seeing them, she was flooded with conflicting thoughts. "Look at that. It's awesome. She is going to have a baby," to "Does she think I'm pregnant?" to "I am so freaking fat. This is so unfair. Why do I have to do this?" all the way over to "I can't wait to be pregnant." She bet not one of those women had to go through what she was going through. How could someone who got pregnant in the usual way ever understand? She felt so sorry for herself, the woman with so many burdens. So many secrets.

She never got used to that waiting room.

The actual ultrasound, though, quickly became a comforting routine. Go in, bladder full, lie in a darkened room while a technician pushed a lubricated probe into your vagina as you stare at a computer screen that shows your ovaries; then, see the doctor, learn that all was going well, egg follicles were developing. Until finally the ultrasounds showed egg follicles that were large and ready to burst open with eggs. And her blood tests showed hormone levels that were perfect for fertilization. It was time. Tur-Kaspa told Amanda to get to Chicago.

## 19

# New Lives

Amanda set off for Chicago on Friday morning, June 4, 2010, alone, in a car packed with her medicine in a cooler. Beside her on the seat were CDs she'd made of her favorite music to help her through the seven-hour drive. She was as prepared as she'd ever be for two weeks that could irrevocably change her life. When she returned she would be pregnant. Or not.

Despite her combination of nervousness and ennui, she could not help noticing the scenery, so different from Hartsville or Charleston or Nashville. She drove past mile upon mile of tender green plants—corn, soybeans, wheat in the black soil that late spring day. When she got to Illinois and saw a field of wind turbines along the side of the highway, she pulled over at a rest stop and walked closer to take a look. She'd never seen wind turbines before. She was dumbstruck by their size and odd resplendence.

Think of the beauty of the land, she told herself. Sometimes it worked for a short while and she was lulled into a sort of trance, driving along the flat straight highway. But then her stubborn thoughts would push themselves to the front of her mind again. This was her way to strike back at GSS. This was her way to destroy the disease so that it would never kill her children. PGD was like a lifeline. That was how she now thought of it.

As she neared Chicago, she grew nervous about the hotel she'd booked. She'd found it online and chosen it because it was cheap and because it was part of a major hotel chain. How bad could it be?

Pretty bad, it turned out. Not that it was dirty, just completely soulless—like a Soviet-era apartment block. The hotel, just off the highway in Skokie, could have been anywhere with its bland appearance. What would she do in that drab place for two weeks? Fortunately, it was clean, and they hadn't forgotten the mini refrigerator she had requested for her medication.

The next morning, she drove to the Reproductive Genetics Institute for her first appointment. Another letdown. She'd built the place up in her mind as the epitome of cutting-edge science, envisioning a clinic housed in a big gleaming modern building in a bustling part of the city. But what she found was a dull brown-brick building on a run-down street. She walked inside. The building's interior was equally depressing, with no attempt to be soothing or attractive, a series of unadorned waiting areas and exam rooms. No warmth here, she thought.

Tur-Kaspa, who'd grown to mythic proportions in her mind, the all-powerful doctor, a serious middle-aged man, was actually very good-looking, she thought, with dark blond hair and dimples. He seemed fully aware of the effect he had on his female patients as he smiled at Amanda and looked into her eyes. And he seemed very sure of himself, almost boastful as he told her of his expertise and the details of the procedure. He did not seem particularly approachable, Amanda thought, but maybe her fear and anticipation were coloring her impressions of the doctor. She reminded herself she was not there to be his best friend.

She called Brad when she left the building. The words rushed out. The hotel. The clinic. Tur-Kaspa. "You can get through it," he told her. "It will be okay."

Amanda called her mother that night; Kathy immediately focused on the hotel. As Amanda described it, dejection in her voice, Kathy cut in. "It sounds really cheap and dingy," she said. "And what about safety?" she asked.

"It's not too bad."

"You're staying two weeks in that room?"

"Yeah."

"I'm coming there," Kathy declared. She hung up and thought again of the enormity of what Amanda was doing, all by herself in Chicago. She knew how emotionally strained her daughter was, she knew how scary the procedure was. She wanted to help Amanda but did not really know how. Going to Chicago was at least a stab at making it easier for her. Money was tight—Buddy had not worked for years and payments to the caregiver she'd needed to keep him at home had eroded their savings. Her job at the free health clinic was not nearly enough to cover their expenses. She'd had to cash in her life insurance to pay for Amanda's wedding, even though that tiny wedding in Jamaica was much cheaper than a big wedding in Hartsville would have been. But Amanda needed her. "I don't care how much it costs," Kathy told herself. "We are going to do something positive and upbeat." She made a plane reservation to come that weekend. She could only stay for the weekend—she had to get back to Hartsville and her job managing the two free medical clinics—which meant she was going to miss the genetic analysis. But she would be there while Amanda anxiously waited to find out which, if any, of Amanda's embryos were surviving and growing.

Kathy had never made peace with Amanda's decision to have PGD. She had prayed over it and accepted that if God did not want this procedure to happen it wouldn't happen. She had to leave it up to God.

And nothing, Kathy vowed, would ever separate her from her children. Amanda is my child, Kathy thought, and I will stand behind her.

After that call to her mother, Amanda spent a restless night in her solitary hotel room, drifting off to sleep, then waking up, looking at the clock by her bedside, drifting off again, waking up. She was in the deep sleep that sometimes comes at the end of a night like that when her cell phone rang. It was a counselor at the genetics institute. The ultrasound showed that her eggs were mature. Tur-Kaspa needed to extract them the next day, before she ovulated. She would need to get Brad to Chicago immediately. They would need his sperm soon after her eggs were extracted from her ovaries.

In an instant her life changed from nervous inaction to nervous activity. Still shaking, she called Brad. "You have to come right away," she told him anxiously. "I'll be there," he replied, telling her that he loved her. They hung up and Amanda stared at the phone. She tried to keep her expectations in check: success was hardly guaranteed. In fact, the odds were against her. Often women had only a few eggs and those eggs failed to be fertilized. Often every egg that was fertilized and developed into an embryo just happened to have the disease gene that the woman was trying to avoid. Embryos that seemed normal and healthy and did not have the disease gene often failed to implant in the woman's uterus.

Brad arrived the next day. He looked around at the dark hotel room, looked out the window at the treeless street. He folded his arms and stared at his wife. "This is it? Jesus, Amanda. This is where you have been staying?"

"Yes," she replied. "I told you."

"Wow, this *is* depressing," he said, shaking his head. But then he caught himself. This was no way to greet his wife. "I would be with you in a heartbeat, if only I could," he told her as he hugged her.

There was no time to waste—Brad had arrived just in time to head off to the genetics institute for the procedure. He was ushered into a small room in an older part of the building to provide a sperm sample. "It's like a sleazy brothel room," he thought when he saw it. The whole thing felt dirty. Afterward, he went to the recovery room to wait for Amanda, struck by the contrast with where he had been. This room had a sterile feel. Functional and clean, but hardly inviting, he thought. He sat nervously in a chair, glanced at his cell phone, tried to read a magazine. He paced a bit. He waited.

Amanda, meanwhile, had been lightly anesthetized and wheeled into a small room where Tur-Kaspa, watching his work on an ultrasound screen, inserted a long needle into each bulging egg sack in her ovaries and sucked out the mature eggs, depositing them into tiny petri dishes filled with a nourishing broth. In less than an hour, Tur-Kaspa was done—he'd retrieved fourteen eggs. His goal had been for Amanda to produce ten to fifteen.

After Amanda woke up, still a bit groggy, Brad drove her back to her hotel and sat next to her bed as she slept some more. He had had only brief interactions with Tur-Kaspa, was not even sure if he would recognize him if he saw him again. The whole thing had felt so impersonal, as if these past few hours, doing the most fraught thing he and Amanda could do, were just part of the routine at the clinic.

Brad watched Amanda sleep as dusk arrived. At about seven o'clock, Brad gently shook her awake.

"Amanda, I have to go to the airport. Will you be okay? I can cancel my flight if you need me."

"You have to go," Amanda replied, turning her head toward him. She understood, she knew he had no choice.

Amanda closed her eyes again, dozing as Brad crept out the door. She awoke the next day to a call from a nurse coordinator at the clinic.

"Amanda," she said. "I have good news. Twelve of the fourteen eggs were successfully fertilized."

Amanda felt a rush of sheer joy.

But then she asked uneasily, "What happened to the other two?"

"They just didn't fertilize," she replied. "That happens in your body all the time."

As soon as she hung up, Amanda called Brad.

"What about the other two?" Brad asked. Then he thought of the twelve. "Oh my God. That is a lot."

That actually was better than average. Tur-Kaspa had told her he expected 70 to 80 percent of mature eggs to fertilize which, in Amanda's case, would have meant about ten or eleven. "But all you need is one good embryo," he told his patients every time.

Still more challenges lay ahead. On average only five of the embryos would grow in those petri dishes—the rest would die. And since each embryo had a fifty-fifty chance of having the GSS mutation, it was entirely possible that every one of the embryos that survived would have the disease gene. And, even if there was an embryo without that mutated gene, the chance that Amanda would get pregnant when Tur-Kaspa implanted it in her uterus was only about 50 percent.

They'd have to wait five days to find out how many embryos survived and grew large enough for the embryologist to safely pluck a couple of cells from each for genetic testing. Meanwhile, Amanda would wait alone in her Skokie hotel, venturing off to a Starbucks to use their free Wi-Fi, bored and anxious, depressed by her lifeless surroundings.

But then Kathy arrived on Friday, taking a cab directly to Amanda's hotel. Her first thought was that she had to get her daughter out of there.

"We are going to stay on the Magnificent Mile and we are going shopping," Kathy told Amanda, knitting her brow as she looked with concern at her daughter. Amanda looked so sad, so dejected. "We are going to have fun," Kathy assured her.

They checked into a Hilton in the heart of the city near Lake Michigan for the weekend. Kathy bought clothes for Amanda. They ate at good restaurants and saw a comedy show at Second City. They even visited the Reproductive Genetics Institute so Kathy could see where the procedures would take place. Kathy observed her daughter observing her. Amanda seemed to be thirsting for an upbeat assessment. What the building looked like wasn't important, Kathy told her. "They are putting their money into what matters, helping couples have children," she reassured her daughter.

Kathy's visit made Amanda realize she did not have to spend her time in her hotel or at the Starbucks nearby. She could go to Chicago and explore the city. Life did not have to be so dreary.

On Monday, she returned to the institute. The embryos were now big enough for the GSS test. The news was good—fortunately, eleven out of twelve had survived. The geneticist planned her strategy. Since no one had ever had PGD for a prion disease, much less GSS, she'd have to make a customized test to look for the mutation. She knew where it was. The prion gene, like every gene in a human cell, is made up of a string of chemical building blocks, the base pairs. The mutation that caused GSS in Amanda's family was 198 base pairs from the start of the prion gene. It was almost incredible to think of the damage that mutation does. Out of the three billion base pairs that make up human DNA, just one was altered. But that one alteration was enough to destroy any human being who inherited it.

The challenge was to find a way to detect that mutation.

She decided to use enzymes that home in on specific sequences in DNA and cut it there, acting like very precise molecular scissors. The GSS gene had one pair of DNA bases that was different from those in the nonmutated gene. She would exploit that difference to look for the GSS gene in the embryos. She would use an enzyme that would only cut the DNA of the gene if that sequence was present. If she did not see that cut, it meant the gene was normal.

The analysis took a day. On Tuesday, Amanda anxiously drove to the brown-brick building, sat in the counseling office on the first floor, and, trying to control her anxiety, looked at the printout the counselor had handed her. The outcome of the genetic testing was textbook perfect: there is a fifty-fifty chance that the child of a parent with GSS will inherit the mutated gene. Of eleven embryos, six had the mutation. The other five were fine.

Amanda stared at the paper with the testing data. Each embryo's result was listed. At that moment, the meaning of what had happened struck her and she could barely breathe. Six of the eleven had been destroyed. She looked at the counselor, who had an elated look on her face. She seemed to be expecting Amanda to be over the moon to have five healthy embryos. But Amanda felt almost strangled by an unbearable sorrow. Those embryos that were discarded could have become her children.

"I passed on a deadly disease to something that could potentially become my child," Amanda thought. And then she had allowed those embryos to be destroyed as if they were meaningless. It was as if she had pointed to them, one by one, and said, "You're sick. You have to go."

As she left the clinic, she started to wail, unable to stifle her cries. She sat on the step outside the clinic, so sad, so bereft, she could not make herself trudge to her car and drive back to her hotel. Six embryos. Six babies. Dead.

But there was little room for this emotion in the clinic. Tur-Kaspa was soon ready to implant an embryo or perhaps two embryos in Amanda's uterus to try to elicit a pregnancy. It had to be done quickly to minimize the time the embryos were living in the artificial environment of a petri dish in an incubator. How many embryos did they want implanted, he asked Amanda. One? Or two?

Amanda and Brad had discussed this and decided they wanted two. They were afraid to take a chance with just one embryo. What if she failed to get pregnant? Their odds, she was certain, were better with two.

Tur-Kaspa looked at her in exasperation. It was her choice, he said. But, he cautioned, she was likely to have twins. She should expect to, in fact.

"No, I won't," Amanda insisted. She was betting on just one of the two making it.

Tur-Kaspa shrugged. Up to her.

The three remaining embryos would be frozen. If the implantation didn't work she could return to Chicago to try again. Or if she did become pregnant and wanted more children in the future she could return and try with one of those frozen embryos.

The next morning, Tur-Kaspa sucked the embryos into a catheter and carefully slid the catheter into Amanda's womb, where he released the embryos. She was staring at the white ceiling above her when she saw a bright light in front of her eyes like a starburst as the embryos struck her uterus. It was as though she'd stared into the sun. The procedure was done.

With a curt "Good luck," Tur-Kaspa strode out of the room.

The next day, on the long drive back to Nashville, Amanda spoke aloud to her unborn babies as she sped down the highway, carrying on a one-way conversation in an attempt to soothe herself.

"It's really important that you stay in there," she told them. "You have to implant because your daddy and I really want you." Every time she crossed a state line she made a video for her unborn babies, saying to them, "Welcome to Indiana," "Welcome to Kentucky," "Welcome to Tennessee." She described what she'd seen in each state, telling them about the wind turbines and telling them she would be really angry and upset with them if they ever made videos while they were driving a car—as she was doing while she drove.

And yet for the entirety of that seven-hour trip, she wondered whether there actually were any babies inside of her.

Eleven days after Tur-Kaspa had implanted the two embryos, Amanda went to Vanderbilt and had her blood drawn for a test that measures levels of the human chorionic gonadotropin hormone, produced by placental cells during pregnancy. Brad ordered the test. Unlike most patients, they wouldn't have to wait for a call from a doctor or nurse to find out the results. They had access to the hospital computer, and lab test results are posted as soon as they are available. Amanda began compulsively checking to see if hers was listed. Finally, later that day, she found it: Her HCG level was 37. A level of 5 means pregnancy and a level that is way above 5 can mean twins. But they were afraid to get their hopes up. Maybe she was not really pregnant or maybe the pregnancy was started but the embryos had recently died and the pregnancy would not last. Or maybe there was a lab error.

Amanda had a second test two days after the first. She and Brad sat down at a hospital computer and pulled up the results. Her HCG level was 272. They waited three days and did the test again. Now the HCG was 819. Brad looked at the computer screen. Then he looked at Amanda and grinned.

"We're having twins," he said.

Amanda smiled back. Buddy's life had ended just as two new lives—two babies without the GSS mutation—were about to begin. It meant something. This, she decided, was a gift of life from her father.

# 20

# Carrying Forth

For so long, Amanda had yearned to be pregnant, lusted for it, envied the women she would see in the parks, in shopping centers, walking down the street, with their protruding pregnant abdomens. She'd wanted to know what it felt like to be pregnant and she wanted babies with all her heart. Now it was happening.

Yet beneath the dizzying euphoria there was always an undercurrent of sadness. Doctors could not predict when her disease would start. Her father's illness had begun when he was forty-eight. Her grandfather's had begun at an extremely late age for GSS—sixty-three. Her great-grandfather had died when he was forty-nine, so his symptoms probably began when he was in his late thirties. Amanda would be twenty-nine when her babies were born. She might not live much beyond their teenage years. They would have to witness the terrible deterioration and death she had seen with her own father. And as soon as they were able to understand, they, like Amanda and Brad, would be nervously waiting for her first symptoms, a trembling hand, a stumble. The thought was always there, in the back of her mind. She was bringing sorrow into the world.

It was a strange, almost unreal time for Amanda, a time when she was in a small world of her own making, isolated, largely left to her own imaginings. She talked to Kathy on the phone; she texted and emailed with Luke; and she spoke to Brad. But otherwise her life contracted—work, sleep, work, sleep. She had no close friends. Almost as soon as she moved to Nashville she'd begun that overwhelming work schedule with little time for anything else.

But there also was another reason for her isolation. She did not want to tell other people—outsiders—her story. Before she'd gotten pregnant, she'd wanted to avoid people pitying her or whispering about her plight. She did not want people discussing among themselves whether it was right to bring those babies into the world. She thought of PGD as her gift to her babies, her way of assuring that they would never have to face what was going to happen to her. She did not want that gift sullied.

It was hard for her to recognize the self she used to be. She remembered her days in Hartsville and in college, filled with friends and family. She'd always been gregarious, outgoing. Friendships had come easily to her. Now she was nearly alone, determined to keep her fears and her fate to herself.

From the start, Amanda's pregnancy was difficult. All the Web sites she consulted said that women are tired for the first few months, yet she could not shake the feeling that what she was experiencing went beyond anything they described. She felt a constant tug of exhaustion as her bleary eyes fought the pull of drowsiness, overcome with a desire to sleep.

Work seemed overwhelming. She was still working twelve-hour nursing shifts, and wondering how much longer she could keep it up. She found herself putting her head down on the table for a quick nap during her lunch break. After work, she trudged up to the apartment door at seven in the evening, was in bed and asleep by eight, not waking until she heard the jarring sound of her alarm at five thirty the next morning.

She called her obstetrician, who was sympathetic but unconcerned. "Well, you are carrying two," she said. Being tired was totally normal. "You have to get through it as best you can."

"Stop working," Brad told her, worried about her health and the health of their babies. He had wanted her to stop as soon as they learned she was pregnant, but he was even more adamant now. He assured her he would find a way to make enough money moonlighting for them to get by. But Amanda could not bring herself to follow his advice. If she stopped working, what would she do? Spend her time in that tiny apartment, alone, letting her emotions take over? Work was a distraction—it was draining, but it also took her out of herself—so she vowed to continue as long as she could.

She had a brief respite from the discomfort of pregnancy at about four months, when it seemed that things were finally on track. She had an ultrasound: they were having a boy and a girl. They set out to choose names. It would be Ava for the girl— ever since she was little Amanda had loved the name Ava, so short and feminine and old-fashioned. Cole for the boy, a more difficult choice but one they agreed on in the end.

A month later, Amanda started having contractions, dull aches like menstrual cramps that would start, then stop, then start again. Her obstetrician said she was not in labor—those contractions were more like muscle spasms, her body was not trying to expel the babies. But by this point, Amanda was ready to stop going in to work. With this twin pregnancy, she was growing enormous, retaining huge amounts of fluid—Amanda ended up gaining ninety pounds of mostly fluid weight. It was wearying.

The next round of contractions started at twenty-nine weeks and they were stronger, more regular, dull, cramping aches deep in her abdomen that happened when her uterus clenched, squeezing like it was trying to push out a baby. Amanda timed them and they were coming at precise intervals, about once every ten minutes. Amanda called her doctor, who told her she had to stay in bed for the rest of her pregnancy. She could get up only to take a shower, use the bathroom, or fix herself something to eat. Amanda's abdomen was so big—her waist grew to fifty inches by thirty-three weeks, more than double its usual circumference—and she was so unwieldy she could only sleep sitting up.

One morning a week later, when she was alone in the apartment and getting dressed. Amanda looked down at her bulbous abdomen and saw a thin red horizontal line, about two and a half inches long, that had formed about an inch above her naval. Her skin was actually splitting. It had stretched so far it had pulled apart. The wound hurt and it bled. She gasped in disbelief. Her skin had stretched to its limit. What would happen if she got even bigger? Impossible to imagine. And that blood oozing from the wound. Was it ever going to stop? Amanda walked over to the medicine cabinet and grabbed a box of Band-Aids. She slid one out of its wrapper and carefully placed it over the wound. Eventually a scab formed, then a scar, a constant reminder.

The contractions continued but never worsened, never got more frequent. The goal now was to keep the babies in her as long as possible. Amanda's doctor gave her Procardia, a blood pressure drug, to help stop preterm labor. If she took a dose of Procardia and still felt another contraction, she was to take a second drug, terbutaline, to relax the uterus. If she still felt contractions, she was to go to the hospital.

A month dragged by. To Amanda's surprise, Tur-Kaspa called a couple of times to check up on her and sent her an e-mail asking her to send photos of the twins after they were born. Old friends from Hartsville kept in touch with occasional calls and Facebook posts. But mostly she relied on phone calls with Kathy, calling her mother nearly every day. "I'm so sorry to be bothering you again," she'd say by way of greeting. She was intensely grateful to her mother for always being there, ready to spend as much time as Amanda needed chatting, consoling, reassuring her.

Amanda wiled away the lonely hours watching movies, reading books, riffling through magazines, and working on a project Kathy gave her to keep her occupied, a baby blanket with the outlines of three giraffes she could embroider with cross-stitch. She was almost always sitting on the couch or in a rocking chair because it was too uncomfortable to lie down. She was plagued by shooting pains from sciatica running from her buttocks down her legs. Brad was terrified that she would go into labor and called every hour to be sure she was not walking around the apartment. "Amanda," he would tell her, "I know you are uncomfortable. I know this is the worst thing you have had to go through. But those babies have to stay in there as long as possible." He brought food home at night so she did not have to get up to prepare dinner. He made lunch for her before he left for work.

Amanda knew it was a risky time but pushed aside any thought that the babies might not make it. She told herself they might come a bit early but they would be okay. She could not let herself peel away the illusion that everything would be fine.

One evening, after Brad had returned home from work, Amanda began having contractions that would not stop. She turned to Brad, fear in her eyes. "I think it's starting," she said. "I am going into labor." Procardia did not help. Terbutaline did not help. She was thirty-three weeks pregnant—seven weeks from when her babies were due. It was much too early for her to have those babies, she thought anxiously. She called her doctor, who told her to take another dose of Procardia and give it fifteen to twenty minutes to work. If the contractions continued, she was to go to the hospital. The drug did not help.

By now the contractions were coming every three minutes and lasting about thirty seconds.

At that stage of pregnancy—thirty-three weeks—most babies survive, but they are at risk for learning and behavioral problems. Most have to spend time in a neonatal intensive care unit before leaving the hospital and have to be taught and coaxed to suck so they can get nourishment.

Terrified, Brad rushed Amanda into their car and sped to the hospital, gripping the steering wheel, his face white with fear. Although both Amanda and Brad worked at Vanderbilt Medical Center, they had chosen Baptist Hospital for the birth. Brad worried that people would peek at Amanda's medical record and see that she had the GSS mutation. They had kept that to themselves—the last thing Brad wanted was sensing his colleagues furtively observing him and Amanda, aware of the difficulty to come in their future. Amanda had a different concern. She just did not want people she knew to peer at her during labor and delivery and see her naked.

Baptist was a better place anyway, she and Brad had told themselves. Its newborn intensive care unit was rated even higher than the unit at Vanderbilt. Yet beneath the excuses she and Brad had given themselves, she also knew that even now, at the culmination of her pregnancy, she had deliberately chosen to be alone.

When Amanda arrived at the hospital, the doctors discovered her blood pressure was dangerously high and her platelet count was dropping. She had a syndrome called HELLP, a very rare variant of preeclampsia. The H is for hemolysis, the breaking down of red blood cells, the EL for elevated liver enzymes and the LP for low platelet count. Blood vessels narrow and vital organs can be deprived of blood. As many as a quarter of pregnant women who develop it die.

"We have to get the babies out of you to save your life," her doctor told her.

Amanda would not—could not—seriously believe her life was in danger. It was too much to take in. As they prepared her for a cesarean delivery, nurses began infusing her with intravenous magnesium to slow her labor. Amanda wept with a terrible guilt as she slipped into a spiral of regret. She had wanted this to happen, she had wished for her pregnancy to end. A part of her knew it was irrational to think that way, but still she had a sense that she had brought this on when she had kept saying to Kathy, to Brad, to herself, that she just wanted the babies to come out.

"The babies will be born tonight," she thought. Nothing is going to prevent that. They might not be okay. They might not even survive. It's too soon. It's much too soon. Tears rolled down her swollen cheeks. Brad, meanwhile, went into his anxious mode, which meant he shut down; he stopped talking and alternately stood silently at Amanda's bedside or paced with his arms crossed, not saying a word.

The nurses told Brad to leave the room and put on a sterile gown, cap, and gloves so he could watch the operation. Meanwhile, Amanda curled up as best she could while a nurse pushed a needle into her spinal canal, injecting a spinal block, a drug that would paralyze her from her lower spine down, preventing all feeling as her doctor cut her open and removed the twins.

Then she lay on her back while the medical staff arranged a barrier in front of her chest to shield her eyes from the operation that was going to take place. Brad returned and stood by Amanda's head. He could see the procedure but only glanced at the surgery once. The rest of the time, he looked at Amanda. Amanda, though, staring at the ceiling, noticed that the huge surgical light overhead was so shiny, she had a blurry view of what was going on. She couldn't not look.

Ava was first to be delivered. Amanda felt a big tug as her doctor pulled the baby out. She felt lighter immediately, and empty. The staff suctioned the infant. A couple of seconds later, Ava cried. Because of the barrier in front of her, Amanda could not see her daughter, but that cry told her the baby was alive. She wept with relief.

"We're going for Cole now," the obstetrician told Amanda. "Cole has dropped down and the cord has wrapped around his neck. We are going to take him out very quickly." She tugged the baby out, but all was silent, no cries. "He's dead," Amanda thought in horror.

"Brad, you have to go to him, you have to check on Cole," she pleaded. Brad ran across the room, his heart pounding as he saw the limp infant, blue from lack of blood. After a few agonizing minutes, Amanda heard Cole whimper. Then the team from the neonatal intensive care unit whisked the infants out of the room, explaining as they dashed off that every minute was precious, that they had to get the babies to intensive care. Amanda never saw them, her view still blocked by that barrier.

Brad stood where the babies had been, paralyzed with fear, frightened for Amanda, frightened for the babies, too frightened to ask questions.

"You should go, be with the babies," Amanda told her husband, and he rushed to catch up with them.

The twins were born on January 18, 2011. Their due date was March 3. Ava weighed four pounds, nine ounces; Cole weighed four pounds, one ounce.

Amanda was wheeled back to her room, desolate. She had to remain hooked up to intravenous magnesium—a vain attempt to stop her labor—for another twenty-four hours. That meant, she was told, she could not see her babies. It did not help much when Brad returned from the nursery and told her that Ava's arm was in a soft cast like a tiny ACE bandage and she had an intravenous line in her head. Cole required oxygen to breathe. Terribly worried, Brad went into his doctor mode, hiding his emotions and speaking dispassionately.

Kathy flew to Nashville immediately, arriving in the morning, and went first to Amanda's room. Before she could even hug her daughter, Amanda pleaded with her to go see the babies. "Please go check on them. Please, Mom, tell me how they are."

Kathy went to the newborn intensive care unit, then rushed back to Amanda's bed, embracing her daughter as Amanda sobbed.

"They are good," she told Amanda, speaking of the babies. "They are doing fine. They are getting excellent care. We will get you in there to see them."

All through that long night in the hospital, Amanda had had time to think, alone in her room, worried about her babies and what was in store for them. "I just hope they will be proud of me," Amanda said to herself. She wanted them to grow up knowing she spared them from inheriting GSS. "They will know I did everything I could do."

Finally, twelve hours after the twins entered the world, Amanda was able to go to the nursery where her babies were staying. A nurse pushed her in a wheelchair, Brad at her side. Kathy was already there, waiting.

The slow procession—Amanda, Brad, and the nurse—entered the NICU. The bigger, healthier babies were at the back of the unit; the tiny sick ones at the front. She saw a tiny baby, eyes fused shut, seemingly no bigger than an orange and covered with downy hair. "Oh my God. Do my babies look like that?" she thought. She averted her eyes. It was too terrifying.

They approached Ava and Cole, who were toward the back, with the more developed and healthier babies. Her first thought, as she peeked into their tiny cribs—little plastic boxes with oval openings—first at Ava and then at Cole, was that they were impossibly small and thin. As she reached in to touch them, tears burned her eyes. They were hooked up to monitors and seemed so fragile; they would need so much care. Their tiny legs poked out of their diapers, which looked as if they'd been made for other, larger, healthier babies. Cole had a clear plastic tube in his nose, a little round white monitor taped to his chest above his heart. Ava lay on her back, arms bent upward as if to say, "Stop. Enough."

But they were alive and they were her children with Brad and they were going to leave that hospital and come home. They were her babies.

Kathy looked at Amanda and her eyes welled with tears. "My courageous daughter accomplished something that meant the world to her," Kathy thought. "These babies do not have it. They do not have the gene for GSS."

As if reading Kathy's thoughts, Amanda looked up from her twins.

"Mom," she said, "It was worth every minute. Everything we've been through. It stopped with me. GSS stopped with me."

# Epilogue

Amanda thinks of GSS as a dark hovering shadow of a figure with glowing red eyes, always there, at the periphery of her vision, biding its time, watching her.

She first saw it that day in her therapist's office, when Geschwind opened the letter and told her she had the mutated gene. She tried to escape, crawling up the back of the couch, trying to claw her way up the wall behind her, letting out a primal scream, then a whimper.

She remembers what her mother and Brad said way back in 2009 when she insisted on being tested for the GSS mutation. Don't do it, they urged her. Don't have that test. And she remembers Geschwind cautioning her: "Once you get that result you can never go back. You had better be sure, absolutely sure, you are ready for it."

We all lose our sense of invulnerability as we grow older but most lose it gradually, over years, over a lifetime. Only a few lose it all at once. For them, nothing is ever the same. The world is instantly cleaved into a before and after, a then and now. With that test result, Amanda had to somehow muster the courage to split off into a different life. How do you learn to do that? She was only twenty-six. She had not had time to have much of an adult life. She looks back on the person she used to be and sees a stranger.

The knowledge has hardened her. In order to cope with what she now knows, a certain part of her had to shut off. If she allows herself to think of it all the time, if she allows her emotions to surface, she will be overcome.

Before she was tested, she thought finding out she had the GSS gene would make her want to live for the moment, would make her, in an odd way, more carefree. Instead, because the knowledge is always there, it brings her down a little bit. That shadowy figure is lurking. She is not as happy as she used to be.

Knowing is exhausting.

But she has also gained perspective.

She no longer reacts to little annoyances, things like being cut off in traffic, a rude remark by a salesperson. Incidents that used to make her flash with anger now seem insignificant.

She is less judgmental. She used to be angry at her sister who decided not to be tested for the gene mutation and went ahead and had another child.

Amanda now accepts her sister's choice, realizing that there is no right or wrong path. She and Holly have grown closer, drawn by their common bond—having children. These days she and Holly send each other e-mails and texts. They call each other. Holly sends Amanda's children Valentine's gifts and she sends them little gifts she finds at Hobby Lobby, an arts and crafts store, for no reason at all—just because she is thinking of them. Before, Amanda felt she and Holly were too different to be close. Now they can talk about their children—though they still avoid the topic of GSS—and enjoy the friendship developing between their kids.

Luke and Amanda remain incredibly close. Luke, now an emergency medicine doctor, married Amanda's childhood friend, Geneva, after reconnecting with her at Amanda's wedding. He and Geneva and their little boy live an hour from

Amanda and Brad and their children. Still, Amanda and Luke manage to get together twice a month.

After Luke married and he and his wife, Geneva, decided to have children, he knew it was time. He would get tested and, if he had the gene, he would use PGD as Amanda had done.

The results came as a shock. Luke received them at home as his father had, but the result was different. He did not have the gene. After checking the letter once more just to make sure he'd read it correctly, he hugged his wife, then walked somberly around the house, feeling alone and surprisingly morose. He called his mother and sobbed; he couldn't bring himself to call Amanda. Kathy insisted that he do it. When Amanda heard the news, she wept with her brother. But she was happy that once again, the disease had been stopped.

After his call with Amanda, Luke called his friend, Tom, a cardiologist, who had taken Luke's blood sample and sent it in for him. The three of them—Luke, Geneva, and Tom—went to a local bar to celebrate. Though it didn't feel like a celebration for the life that had just been handed back to him—it felt more like a funeral. Luke was overwhelmed by waves of grief for those in his family who hadn't been spared, and guilt for his own good fortune. He would gradually come to terms with his fate and rejoice at his incredible good luck, but his relief remained always bittersweet.

Inevitably, the years of struggle have weighed on Amanda and Brad. People who go through serious medical issues aren't spared the usual trials of marriage. There were moments when one or the other would cry out, "Why did we even start all this?" There were times when their love for each other became background noise to the problems in their lives. They had always promised each other they would never let that happen, but somehow it did. But they came through the stressful times. Even when their problems almost got the better of them, they prevailed. They no longer fight the angry emotions that sometimes make their marriage difficult—they make space for them because they have learned they are not going away. But they are also buoyed by their intense bond, a feeling they can get through what comes to them, a hard-earned conviction based on the traumas they have weathered already.

They have three children now. When the twins were two, Brad and Amanda returned to Chicago and used one of the remaining frozen embryos to have another baby, a little boy named Tatum. Every day with those children has to be special, Amanda feels. It is a taxing way to live, but she can't stop herself. She knows she will die from GSS and she thinks she has a good idea when. Scientists would say her ideas about timing are hunches not grounded in rigorous data, but she has convinced herself. Her father started getting sick in his fifties. She thinks she will start noticing symptoms when she is in her early forties, when the twins are barely teenagers. GSS will come earlier for her, she is convinced, believing the stress of her knowledge will speed up the disease. It came later for her dad, who lived in blissful ignorance until GSS was upon him.

But this demanding knowledge has also led her to continue her participation in research that might one day lead to a cure. For one study, she offered her skin cells to researchers attempting to turn abnormal prion proteins into normal ones. And through the CJD Foundation, the advocacy group for people who have prion diseases, she got to know leading scientists in the field and began following studies that give her hope for her own future. Some avenues look especially promising—one approach uses proteins that attach themselves to prions, freezing them in their normal shapes so they cannot become misshapen and cause disease. The CJD Foundation also calls on her to talk to couples contemplating having PGD and to doctors whose patients have prion diseases and want to know their options for having children. She feels she is helping others and that is a powerful motivation.

When she was in Nashville, saving for PGD, she felt overwhelmed by raw emotion, afraid to make friends, unwilling to tell people what she was going through. Now, living in Charleston where Brad is in practice, she is much more open about her genetic fate. She never just blurts it out to new acquaintances. Instead, she lets the subject come up naturally, talking to another mother, for example.

"Oh, you have twins. Do twins run in your family?"

"Yes, my husband is a twin."

"Then you must have expected it."

"No, actually, I had in vitro fertilization."

"Did you have a fertility problem?"

"No, I have a genetic condition."

Brad has tried to avoid dwelling on what is to come, hoping to cherish the time they have left, but Amanda is still the obsessive planner she always has been. She thinks incessantly about how to prepare her children and hopes to bring up GSS naturally with them, answering questions as they arise rather than planning a day when she sits them down for The Talk. But she has alluded to her death. When Ava and Cole were three, she said to them, "Before Mommy leaves this world we are going to go to Africa together and we are going to stand on the bridge over Victoria Falls. We are going to do that together."

Ava clings to that story, asking Amanda repeatedly, "Mommy, what are we going to do before you die?"

Meanwhile, she is preparing a legacy for them. Every year, on each child's birthday, she makes a video telling the child what she and the three children have done, what new things the child is doing that she just loves, and what the child is doing that she just can't stand. She discusses what is happening in prion research. She talks about life in general, about her life. Then she saves the video as a vivid memory of the days when she was young and healthy. She does not want her children's enduring visions of her to be a woman bent over in a wheelchair, unable to talk, unable to communicate, writhing in pain. If there is one thing she wants them to remember about her, it is the depths of her love for them.

She is also fighting this fight for her father. He was so angry at GSS, so passionate about finding out what to do about it so his family would not have to be afflicted. What she has done, she tells herself, having children without the gene mutation, helping other people through the CJD Foundation, loving Brad and making a life with him, is, in her way, saying to GSS, "Fuck off, go shove it," for her dad.

Buddy would have smiled at that, she thinks.

Then he would have said, "Don't talk like that."

# Notes

## PROLOGUE

9. *They called it kuru—"to be afraid" or "to shiver"*: D. C. Gajdusek and V. Zigas, "Degenerative Disease of the Central Nervous System in New Guinea—the Endemic Occurrence of Kuru in the Native population," *New England Journal of Medicine*, November 14, 1957, v. 257, 974.

9. *It was identified by its early symptoms*: Ibid.

9. *No one had ever been known to recover from kuru*: Ibid., 975.

9. *it was found only among The Fore*: Ibid., 977.

9. *They thought the disease was caused by sorcery*: Judith Farquhar and D. Carleton Gajdusek, *Kuru. Early Letters and Field Notes from the Collection of D. Carleton Gajdusek* (New York: Raven Press, 1981), 286-288.

9. *The Fore population, about ten thousand individuals*: Ibid., 977.

10. *The men—who subsisted primarily on the animals they hunted*: Robert Klitzman, *The Trembling Mountain. A Personal Account of Kuru, Cannibals, and Mad Cow Disease* (Boston: Perseus Publishing, 1998).

10. *The surrounding peoples had pushed*: Ibid., 21.

10. *the only time in known history*: Ibid., 41.

## CHAPTER 2

27. *The brain arrived in the mail*: Judith Farquhar and D. Carleton Gajdusek, *Kuru. Early Letters and Field Notes from the Collection of D. Carleton Gajdusek* (New York: Raven Press, 1981), xxiii.

27. *But when the scientists did the usual tests*: Ibid., and Vincent Zigas, *Laughing Death: The Untold Story of Kuru* (Clifton, NJ: Humana Press, 1990), 224-225.

27. *He decided to make a last-minute detour*: Ibid.

28. *"Gajdusek is not authorized"*: Ibid., 26–27.

28. *Gajdusek was already on his way*: Ibid.

28. *their diet was made up of*: Ibid., 227.

29. *Zigas thought Gajdusek was "one of those globetrotters"*: Zigas, *Laughing Death*, 226.

29. *meaningless diagnoses of diseases*: Ibid., 23.

29. *had become addicted*: Ibid., 21.

29. *treated the diseases that were treatable*: Ibid., 256.

30. *Gajdusek described their "fixed and pained faces"*: Farquhar and Gajdusek, *Kuru*, 12.

30. *Like the women, the child could not walk*: Ibid., 11.

30. *"I looked at those kids"*: *The Genius and the Boys*, documentary film directed by Bosse Lindquist (2009).

30. *"is so astonishing an illness"*: Farquhar and Gajdusek, *Kuru*, 8.

31. *One of Gajdusek's guides*: Ibid.,143.

31. *Gajdusek himself was tortured*: Ibid.

32. *"This is what I felt when I first met Carleton"*: Klitzman, *The Trembling Mountain*, 17.

32. *At age ten, Gajdusek stenciled the names*: D. Carleton Gajdusek, "Biography for the Nobel Prize in Medicine," 1976, www.nobelprize.org/nobel_prizes /medicine/laureates/1976/gajdusek-bio.html.

32. *Gajdusek sought children with kuru*: Farquhar and Gajdusek, *Kuru*, 11.

32. *he began bringing dozens of young boys*: AP, "Nobel Laureate is Accused of Child Abuse," *The New York Times*, April 6, 1966.

32. *there were no formal adoption papers:* Ibid.

32. *Fore children adored him*: Zigas, *Laughing Death*, 231.

33. *Gajdusek began to review the possible causes*: Gajdusek and Zigas, "Degenerative Disease of the Central Nervous System in New Guinea, 976-977.

33. *He'd be safe, he told himself*: Zigas, *Laughing Death*, 237.

33. *try, in a hit-or-miss way*, Farquhar and Gajdusek, *Kuru*, 16.

33. *Next, they gave another group*: Ibid., 27.

34. *Gajdusek sent a pleading letter*: Ibid., 14.

34. *Gajdusek even requested to have two girls*: Ibid., 15.

34. *"Most important now is haste"*: Ibid.

34. *Kuru had first appeared among the Fore*: Ibid., 293.

35. *A full two-thirds of the* children: Gajdusek and Zigas, "Degenerative Disease of the Central Nervous System in New Guinea," 975.

35. *Fore men typically got protein:* Farquhar and Gajdusek, *Kuru,*171, 227.

35. *They found nothing unusual:* Gajdusek and Zigas, "Degenerative Disease of the Central Nervous System in New Guinea," 978.

35. *"mighty unusual to explain why":* Ibid.

35. *"What is urgently needed":* Farquhar and Gajdusek, *Kuru,* 14–15.

36. *"We got the 'dastardly deed' done":* Ibid., 57.

36. *The brain was full of holes:* Ibid., 112–13.

37. *Those files, Gajdusek boasted:* Farquhar and Gajdusek, *Kuru,* 101.

37. *"please urge the NEJM to get our paper out":* Ibid., 95.

37. *It described the disease in the patients:* Gajdusek and Zigas, "Degenerative Disease of the Central Nervous System in New Guinea," 974–978.

38. *"The closest condition I can think of":* Farquhar and Gajdusek, *Kuru,* 155.

38. *CJD had first been described in 1920:* Wolfgang G. May, "Creutzfeld-Jakob Disease," *Acta Neurologica Scandinavia,* 1968, v. 44, 1.

39. *He wrote to E. Graeme Robertson, a pathologist:* Farquhar and Gajdusek, *Kuru,* 273.

39. *He received a letter from an American veterinarian:* Richard Rhodes, *Deadly Feasts: Tracking the Secrets of a Terrifying New Plague* (New York: Simon & Schuster, 1997), 46.

40. *At the suggestion of a friend, Hadlow had visited:* William J. Hadlow, "Kuru Likened to Scrapie: The Story Remembered," *Philosophical Transactions of the Royal Society of London B,* 1959, v. 1510, 3644.

40. *Hadlow published his observations:*W. J. Hadlow, "Scrapie and Kuru," *The Lancet,* 1959, v. 274, 289–290.

40. *Hadlow called the thus far undetectable scrapie agent:* Ibid.

40. *Gajdusek, who had never heard of scrapie:* Beat Hornlimann, Detlev Reisner, Hans A. Kretzschmar, eds., *Prions in Humans and Animals* (Berlin: De Gruyter, 2009), 40.

41. *anesthetized and inoculated a chimpanzee:* Rhodes, *Deadly Feasts,* 71.

42. *But his attempts to transmit:* D. Carleton Gajdusek, "Unconventional Viruses and the Origin and Disappearance of Kuru", *Science,* 1977, v. 197, 948.

43. *Gerstmann presented the case:* Colin A. Masters, D. Carleton Gajdusek and Clarence J. Gibbs, Jr., "Isolations from the Gerstmann-Straussler Syndrome with an Analysis of the Various Forms of Amyloid Plaque Deposition in the Virus Induced Spongiformencephalopathies," *Brain,* 1981, v. 104, 560.

44. *Later, in 1936, after Berta H. died:* J. Gerstmann, E. Straussler, I. Scheinker,

"Uber eine eigenartige hereditar-familiare erkrankung des zentralnervensystems Zugliech ein Beitrag zur frage des vorzeitigen lokalen alterns," Z Neurol, 1936, v. 154, 636-762.

44. *"These formations are shapes that are rarely found"*: Masters, Gajdusek, and Gibbs, Jr., "Isolations from the Gerstmann-Straussler Syndrome," *Brain*, 1981, v. 104, pp. 561-562.

44. *the average age of death was forty-six*: Ibid., 562.

44. *researchers traced the original family's illness*: Hornlimann, Riesner, Kretzschmar, eds., *Prions in Humans and Animals*, 210-212.

## CHAPTER 5

69. *finally, in 1982, he had published the article*: S. B. Prusiner, "Novel Proteinaceous Infectious Particles Cause Scrapie," *Science*, April 9, 1982, v. 216, 136-144.

70. *discovery that enzymes that chew away at proteins*: Stanley B. Prusiner, *Madness and Memory: The Discovery of Prions—A New Biological Principle of Disease* (New Haven: Yale University Press, 2014), 86-90

70. *"beginning to resemble science fiction"*: Ibid. 90-91.

71. *He'd taken to heart advice he'd been given by Frank Westheimer*: Ibid, 85.

71. *he hit upon a good one*: Ibid., 93.

71. *He said it out loud, PREE-on*: Ibid., 86-87.

72. *Even the term "prion" irritated that reviewer*: Ibid., 89-91.

73. *A better name for "prions," he suggested, might be "dorothies"*: Ibid., 93.

73. *Prusiner was stung by the reaction*: Ibid., 1.

73. *he would call it a "hardon"*: Personal communication with the author.

73. *theorizing that perhaps the mysterious "scrapie agent"*: Prusiner, *Madness and Memory*, 113-114.

74. *"The implications of the findings may be enormous"*: Lawrence K. Altman, "Substance Tied to Alzheimer's in Coast Study," *The New York Times*, December 7, 1983.

74. *he "would be more cautious"*: Ibid.

74. *Glenner further wounded Prusiner*: Ibid., 115.

75. *"ran counter to all of the basic tenets"*: Charles Weissman, personal communication with the author.

76. *in 1987, a forty-one-year-old man came to the University of California*: Prusiner, *Madness and Memory*, 155.

76. *Bruce Miller, a neurologist*: Ibid.

76. *an autopsy revealed she had had GSS*: Ibid.

77. *And, though she had never before even held a pipette*: Karen Hsiao, personal communication with the author.

77. *"I want to work in your lab"*: Ibid.

77. *In July 1986*: Ibid.

78. *She rushed back and forth*: Ibid.

79. *in 1984, when a twenty-nine-year-old woman called him*: Thomas Bird, personal communication with the author.

79. *She sent Bird a four-page handwritten letter*, Ibid.

79. *They called family members and contacted the cousins*: Ibid.

79. *That man died two years later, in 1986*: Ibid.

80. *They called Colin Masters*: Ibid.

80. *In August 1987, he wrote to Bird*: Ibid.

80. *Bird sent Hsiao DNA from the blood*: Ibid.

81. *Only one wanted to know. He tested positive*: Thomas Bird, personal communication with the author.

81. *She was at home when she got the call*: Karen Hsiao, personal communication with the author.

81. *Prusiner surprised Hsiao by giving her a hug*: Ibid.

81. *He published this paper in* Nature: Karen Hsiao, et al., "Mutant prion proteins in Gerstmann-Straussler-Scheinker disease with neurofibrillary tangles," *Nature Genetics*, 1992, v. 1, 68-71.

82. *in 1990, Weissmann thought of an experiment*, Prusiner, *Madness and Memory*, 176-177.

82. *"Stan, everything is working out your way"*: Ibid., 177-179.

83. *He began imagining spending the next thirty or forty years*: Ibid., 214.

83. *In early 1996, Prusiner got a call*: Ibid., 190.

84. *The F.B.I, as it turned out*: "Nobel Laureate is accused of child abuse," *The New York Times*, April 6, 1996.

84. *In one instance, he wrote that boys*: *The Times Higher Education*, November 15, 1996 (www.timeshighereducation.com/news/a-laureate-accused/91481.article).

85. *"I am one," Gajdusek replied*: "Nobel Laureate is accused of child abuse," *The New York Times*, April 6, 1996.

85. *one of the scientists who had put up his house*: Robert Gallo, personal communication with the author.

85. *At 5:00 a.m. the phone rang*: Prusiner, *Madness and Memory*, 218.

85. *But,* Science *also reported*: Gretchen Vogel, "Prusiner Recognized for Once Heretical Prion Theory," *Science*, 1997, v. 278, 214.

## CHAPTER 16

191. *The tone was set in the 1960s*: Gina Kolata, "Robert G. Edwards Dies at 87; Changed Rules of Conception with First 'Test Tube Baby,'" *New York Times*, April 11, 2013, page A1.

191. *For nine years, Edwards traveled*: Ibid.

192. *But, finally one doctor, Molly Rose*: Robert G. Edwards, "The bumpy road to human *in vitro* fertilization," *Nature Genetics*, October 10, 2001, 1091.

193. *In 1972, they succeeded*: Ibid., 1092.

193. *It took two years*: Ibid., 1093.

193. *Edwards and Steptoe tried more than a hundred times*: Kolata, "Robert G. Edwards Dies at 87," *New York Times*, April 11, 2013, A1.

193. *Lesley Brown, who had previously tried for nine years*: Ibid.

193. *On July 26, 1978, Brown was ready*: Ibid.

194. *now they have pregnancy rates of 70 to 80 percent*: Centers for Disease Control and Prevention, "Assisted Reproductive Technology National Summary Report Figures," www.cdc.gov/art/reports/2013/national-summary-figures.html.

194. *Verlinsky called a group of experts together*: Personal communication with the author from Dr. Ilan Tur-Kaspa and Richard Rawlins, professor emeritus of Obstetrics and Gynecology at Rush University Medical Center, Chicago.

195. *"It's pretty much true that anything"*: Personal communication between the author and Dr. James Grifo.

195. *For all their bravado*: Ibid.

195. *of the first ten women who came to Tur-Kaspa*: Personal communication between the author and Dr. Ilan Tur-Kaspa.

196. *1 to 2 percent error rate*: Personal communication between the author and Svetlana Rechitsky, embryologist at Verlinsky's center when Amanda went there.

# Acknowledgments

When I began this book, the Baxleys were strangers to me, and I to them. But they opened their lives, patiently answering questions that forced them to relive some of the most painful experiences possible. They sent me photos and videos of doctor visits. They invited me into their homes. And they told me a story that I found deeply moving and inspiring. It is almost impossible to fully express my gratitude for their cooperation and trust. I am especially grateful to Amanda, Kathy, and Tim, whose generosity had no bounds. I also owe a huge debt to the others, Brad, Mike, Merle, and Billy's family—his daughter, Jennifer, his son, Davis, and his partner, Steve Wood—who were incredibly helpful and forthright as I asked question after probing question. They touched my heart.

I also want to acknowledge Michael Geschwind of the University of California in San Francisco and Thomas Bird of the University of Washington, who helped me learn the science of prion diseases and sent me journal articles on pertinent studies. I also want to thank the many scientists who answered my questions and provided useful data: Robert Klitzman of Columbia University, Paul Brown of the National Institutes of Health, Karen Hsiao Ashe of the University of Minnesota, and Colin Masters of the University of Melbourne. David Housman of MIT helped me understand some complex molecular biology, and Murali Doraiswamy of Duke University alerted me to a journal article about Amanda's PGD that inspired my *New York Times* article that led to this book. The CJD Foundation welcomed me to a family conference that had traditionally barred outsiders and to them, too, I am grateful.

My husband, Bill, was, as always, supportive and patient, a willing reader of draft after draft of my manuscript. My friend Jane McCallister read my near-final manuscript overnight and pointed out that the prologue gave too much away. My agent, Katinka Matson of Brockman, Inc., realized that my *Times* article could be a book and urged me to pursue it.

Finally, I am truly grateful to my gifted editor, Tim Bartlett, executive editor at St. Martin's Press, who acquired the book and helped shape it from the outset. He saw what this book could be and made it what it is. I also want to acknowledge skilled and insightful editing by Nell Casey, a freelance editor, whose help in the final stages was invaluable.

Tim Bartlett's assistants at St. Martin's Press, Claire Lampen and Annabella Hochschild, were extremely helpful and Claire, in particular, provided useful comments on the initial drafts of my manuscript. Finally, I want to acknowledge early champions of the book at St. Martin's: Sally Richardson, George Witte, and Dori Weintraub.

.

Dear Reader: Thank you for reading *Mercies in Disguise*. There are few families like the Baxleys who would be willing to relive the most terrible days of their lives in order to tell us the story of what it is like to live with GSS. I am humbled by their bravery and honesty and am left fervently wishing there were better answers for people with prion diseases. I hope you are as moved as I am and that you, like me, want to find a way to help. I found out that by making a small donation to prion disease research through the CJD Foundation (http://cjdfoundation.org/mercies), we can help make a difference for all those who suffer from this devastating group of diseases.

With best wishes,
Gina Kolata

# Index

BB = William H. "Bill" Baxley, Jr.

1. What is the meaning of the title, *Mercies in Disguise*? What mercies are apparent for the family members? Do the family members see different mercies?

2. If you knew that you were at risk for a fatal genetic condition that had no cure, would you want to be tested for the genetic mutation? Why or why not? What if the person at risk were your child? Your spouse?

3. Why do you think the history of the Fore in New Guinea was included? How did the discovery of kuru lay a foundation for discoveries about GSS and other prion diseases?

*Discussion Questions*

4. What role do chance or coincidence play in scientific discoveries discussed in the book? What role does scientific collaboration play?

5. What role did each member of the family (Tim, Mike, Buddy, and the others) play in uncovering the diagnosis? Would they have been likely to find a diagnosis without this collaboration?

6. Why was it so difficult to obtain a diagnosis, even in a family with medical backgrounds and with access to expert neurologists?

7. How does knowing that they have the mutation affect some of the individuals in the book? Are there unexpected consequences from knowing their diagnosis? How are individuals who learn they do not have the mutation affected by that knowledge?

8. How do you feel about the choice of a family member who opts not to be tested? Can you understand their POV?

St. Martin's Griffin

9. Each individual makes their own decision to pursue genetic testing. How much do religious views versus scientific knowledge impact their decision? Are religious views necessarily at odds with scientific mind views?

10. How does our increasing ability to test for genetic illnesses before they occur affect your views on the importance of protecting the privacy of medical records?

11. How did Bill Baxley, Sr.'s, experience with the disease differ from that of his sons? Did knowing the name of the disease affect Billy and Buddy's hope as the illness progressed?

12. Why did Amanda's mother, Kathy, ask her to wait to be tested until after her father had died?

13. Do you believe her father, Buddy, wanted her to be tested? Why or why not?

14. Which Baxley family member did you find yourself relating to the most? Why?